The Complete Idiot's Reference Card for Teens

The Four Steps to Changing Your Looks

1. Decide what goals you want to achieve.
2. Figure out the right steps to take to get there.
3. Take those right steps.
4. Celebrate your success—at every step of the process.

Five Steps to Eating Well and Feeling Great

1. Pay attention to what you eat.
2. Understand what makes a good, nutritious diet, and try to choose healthy, balanced food most of the time.
3. Get close to nature! (At least in what you eat.)
4. Enjoy your food.
5. Eat when you're hungry; stop eating when you're full.

Tips for Exercising Safely

- ✧ Respect your body's messages. Know when to slow down and when to stop.
- ✧ Balance your muscles, balance your program.
- ✧ Train by knowing—and pushing—the limits.
- ✧ Care for your feet.
- ✧ Keep the impact low.
- ✧ Use good form and learn proper technique.
- ✧ Combine exercise with eating well and getting adequate rest.
- ✧ Always warm up and cool down.
- ✧ Stay hydrated.

alpha books

Gym Etiquette—Tips for Keeping Your Gym Friends

- ✧ Watch first; observe the traffic pattern so you can blend in and not get in anybody's way.
- ✧ Don't hog the machines.
- ✧ Don't lift right near the dumbbell rack.
- ✧ Put your equipment back when you're done.
- ✧ Wipe down the machines after you use them.

Stretching Tips

- ✧ Wear loose, unbinding clothes.
- ✧ Warm up before stretching.
- ✧ Stretch slowly to where you feel slow tension—but *not* pain.
- ✧ Don't bounce.
- ✧ Hold each stretch 30 to 60 seconds.
- ✧ Do each stretch three times.

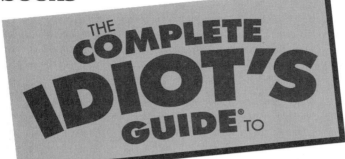

THE COMPLETE IDIOT'S GUIDE® TO

Looking Great
for *Teens*

by Ericka Lutz

Macmillan USA, Inc.
201 West 103rd Street
Indianapolis, IN 46290

A Pearson Education Company

12746665

Copyright © 2001 by Ericka Lutz

THE COMPLETE IDIOT'S GUIDE TO and Design are registered trademarks of Macmillan USA, Inc.

International Standard Book Number: 0-02-863985-5
Library of Congress Catalog Card Number: Available upon request.

03   02   01   8   7   6   5   4   3   2   1

Interpretation of the printing code: The rightmost number of the first series of numbers is the year of the book's printing; the rightmost number of the second series of numbers is the number of the book's printing. For example, a printing code of 01-1 shows that the first printing occurred in 2001.

Printed in the United States of America

Publisher
Marie Butler-Knight

Product Manager
Phil Kitchel

Managing Editor
Cari Luna

Senior Acquisitions Editor
Randy Ladenheim-Gil

Development Editor
Jennifer Moore

Senior Production Editor
Christy Wagner

Copy Editor
Rachel Lopez

Illustrator
Jody Schaeffer

Cover Designers
Mike Freeland
Kevin Spear

Book Designers
Scott Cook and Amy Adams of DesignLab

Indexer
Amy Lawrence

Layout/Proofreading
Steve Geiselman
Mary Hunt

Contents at a Glance

Contents

Foreword

We've all heard those old expressions "beauty is only skin-deep" and "beauty comes from the inside." While these are certainly true, it's also a fact that we all want to look our best. This is especially true of teens, who might not know how to deal with the many changes their bodies, hair, and skin are going through.

I've been in the beauty business for 10 years now, and I've learned many secrets on how to look my best from the top professional hair-stylists, makeup artists, nutritionists, personal trainers, and exercise instructors I've worked with. But back when I was a teenager in Peoria, Illinois, I was clueless about nutrition; exercise; how to take care of my skin, hair, and nails; and how to apply makeup in a way that complemented my looks.

I had no idea eating hamburgers and French fries every day could affect my body, mood, and energy level. I believed if I bought the shampoo and conditioner I saw advertised in all the magazines, my hair would look great. I would go nuts in the makeup aisle of the drugstore, thinking the more makeup I bought and slathered on, the better I would look, even if it meant wearing hideous blue eye shadow and fuchsia lipstick—together! I thought the same weight-lifting program my football-playing brothers followed was the right one for me. Only after years of cold, hard experience did I realize that eating properly was essential for feeling and looking my best; that I needed to choose skin and hair care products and makeup suited to my hair, skin type, and coloring; and that exercise wasn't a one-size-fits-all proposition.

Also, when I was a teenager, I was more interested in trying to look like all the people I saw in magazines and on television. It wasn't until much later that I realized that I should be trying to look my personal best, instead of a bad imitation of someone else.

That's why I was so happy to discover *The Complete Idiot's Guide to Looking Great for Teens*. I really wish I had had this book when I was a teen. It would have saved me from making a lot of scary mistakes. Its sensible, up-to-date, easily accessible advice would have made those difficult years a lot easier. (And actually, it contains tons of information that is just as relevant for adults, which is why I'm keeping this book on a shelf where I can reach for it quickly whenever I have a question.)

I also like that this book is written to each individual teen, and that it encourages everyone to look their best without conforming to someone else's standard. Regardless of what your beauty goals are, *The Complete Idiot's Guide to Looking Great for Teens* will give you healthy, safe, easy-to-follow tips on improving your looks.

As the author of *The Complete Idiot's Guide to Being a Model* and the host of the Elite Model Search for several years, I've spoken to thousands of teens. Almost all of them have asked me questions about health, beauty, and nutrition, so I know how necessary a book like this is. I think all teens will love *The Complete Idiot's Guide to Looking Great for Teens* because it covers all the issues relevant to their lives, it provides the information they're looking for, and it speaks to them in their own language. This is a must-read for every young person.

Roshumba Williams

Supermodel Roshumba Williams has graced the covers and pages of *Vogue, Harper's Bazaar, Elle, Top Model, Cosmopolitan, Allure,* and *Time Out New York.* She has modeled for many top designers, including Yves Saint Laurent, Christian Dior, Chanel, Versace, Armani, and Anne Klein. For four years, Roshumba stood out as one of the few African-American women to establish herself as a model for the *Sports Illustrated* Swimsuit Edition. Roshumba has also added television and movies to her resumé. She is seen daily on VH1, where she hosts regular programming and high-profile specials. She also appeared in the Woody Allen film *Celebrity*, and has a recurring role as Qali in the *Mortal Kombat* TV series.

Introduction

Walk the aisles of any bookstore and you'll see a lot of health and beauty books for sale, but most of them aren't specifically for teens. This one is! It's a book about looking great. It's also a book about feeling great, since …

✧ What you think and feel affects how you look.

✧ How you look affects how you think and feel.

This book is for teens who want to make changes in how they look and feel. Simple as that, Jack.

If you're like most teens, you want to look great, and you're concerned about health. You also know a lot already. You've spent years subjected to gym classes, lectures on eating good food, and all those posters of the food pyramid hanging on classroom walls. Teens know they should exercise, and they know a lot about nutrition:

✧ Ninety-eight percent understand the importance of eating plenty of fruits, vegetables, and high-fiber foods.

✧ Eighty percent can name at least three of the five food groups.

✧ Sixty-five percent say eating habits can affect future health.

But do teens actually eat well and exercise enough? Not really. If you want to learn more about food and exercise, and if you want to learn more about the "outside" parts of looking great—your hair, your smile, your weight, your style—this book's for you.

Looking Great, Feeling Great

You're no idiot, of course! You know you're smart, but sometimes you think everybody knows more than you do. The best part about this book is it's basic. That means if you already know something about a particular subject, my explanations might seem dumb or too simple. But at other places in the book, you'll appreciate the explanations. It's a beginner, baby-step book that breaks it all down. Because sometimes, you just gotta start from scratch, Baby.

What's in the Book?

The Complete Idiot's Guide to Looking Great for Teens is divided into sections. Each section covers a basic area of looking great, and each of these sections has specific chapters that focus in on things you want to—and need to—know about looking terrif. Here's what's up in each section:

Part 1, "Working Toward Your Ideal Body and Look": You're not gonna get somebody else's body (the technology's not that advanced yet). So it's a question of learning to live with—and love—your own. No, not as it is—this is a book about changing, right? In Chapter 1, "Your Life in the Teen Machine," you'll think about where you are now, and what kinds of things have influenced your self-image. In Chapter 2, "Improvement!? You're Not Out to Lunch," you'll identify your goals and hopes for the future, and figure out how to work those changes into your busy life.

Part 2, "Healthy Eating": Food is your fuel, but it does more than just make your body go; it determines a great deal of how you feel and look. In Chapter 3, "Balanced Diet 101—Teen Style," we'll look at some nutrition nitty gritty. The real deal about how specific foods make you look and feel. Chapter 4, "Eating on the Run—Eating for Your Lifestyle," focuses on food and the teen lifestyle. What's the basic eating plan? We'll look at breakfast, lunch, dinner, snacks, mall food, food for staying awake with, and food to fall asleep by. Chapter 5, "Changes and Choices in Food," is all about specific ways to change your eating. That means we'll cover shopping, cooking, and vegetarianism, too.

Part 3, "Safe and Effective Weight Loss": Dieting isn't healthy for teens; but, at the same time, teens are tremendously concerned about weight. This section is all about fat—and thin. In Chapter 6, "Fat and Thin—Trimming the Shape You're In," we'll look at ways to trim up safely. And Chapter 7, "Help and Maintenance," emphasizes the "don'ts" and what to do if you're stuck and stressing on your weight. This is where to turn if you need help with food and eating issues.

Part 4, "Work That Body! Safe Fitness for Teens": Diet is only a piece of the "Looking Great" puzzle. Moving that body makes a big difference, too. In this jumbo section, you'll learn about exercise—in general, and in particular. Chapter 8, "Setting Up and Exercisin' It!" talks about ways to exercise safely and have fun doing it, how to get ready to exercise, and the inside scoop on getting the gear. Chapter 9, "Life at the Gym," takes you inside the gym. Chapter 10, "Outside Exercise and Team Sports," takes you outside (interested in walking, running, biking?) for your workout. Chapter 11, "Home Base—Working Out at Home," is for the broke and lazy—ways to work out without leaving the house. In Chapter 12, "Martial Arts—Far Eastern–Style Fitness," it's "Hai YAH!" time—from Aikido to

Karate, life on the mat. And in Chapter 13, "Dance—Finding Your Rhythm," learn what you need to know before you strap on those tap shoes, pull up those tights, and start to move that bod.

Part 5, "Looking Good—from the Outside In": Nutrition and exercise are vital to looking great. But, frankly, so is skin care, hair care, and fashion. In this section, it's about the surfaces. Chapter 14, "The Skin You're In," is all about skin, the body's largest organ. Chapter 15, "Looking Great—Hair and Grooming," is about hair—washing it, cutting it, styling it—and teeth and nails, too. And Chapter 16, "Working on Your Image, Style, and Makeup," which is all about image and style, gives you tips on style, shopping, and make-up to make your coolest self-image come alive on the outside.

Part 6, "Dealing with the Uglies": It's hard to find balance and moderation in life. These final two chapters, Chapters 17 and 18, teach ways to get it—and keep it—together, especially when things get rough. Chapter 17, "Attack of the Hormones!" focuses on ... you got it ... hormones. And Chapter 18, "Stress Busting," is all about reducing stress.

And in the back of the book, don't forget to check out the appendix for more excellent, insightful, and useful info (I hope, I hope!).

Those Cute Little Boxes

Aside from the basic words on each page, you'll also notice some info in little boxes. What's up with that?

PHAT Fact

Just the facts, ma'am! Well, also some tips and trivia about diet, fitness, health, beauty, and whatever else is on my mind.

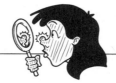

Beautiful? NOT!

Whoa! Watch out! This is the *warning!* box. It gives you the red light ("Will you cut that out!?!?!?").

He Sez

Quotes from guys. What does he think about the issue?

She Sez

Quotes from girls. What's she got to say?

I'm Not Trying to Be Sexist!

Language is really tricky; Hey, I gotta let you know that sometimes I use "he" when I mean "he or she" or I use "her" when I mean "him or her." I try to alternate. This book is for everybody and, unless I'm talking about jock straps or periods, I'm usually talking about both sexes. I also use the terms "guys" and "girls" because those are the terms most teens I know use—if you wanna say "grrls," that's cool by me, too.

So Don't *Sue Me!*

... I'm not a doctor or a lawyer. Just want to let you know that I'm doing the best I can, and I'm fact-checking with the experts as best I can. But I'm not liable. Check with your doctor, your coach, and your parents before following my advice, Babe!

Acknowledgments

I leaned pretty heavy on some people while writing this book, and they get extra special credit: my loving Sweet Matoogie Bill and Ms. Annie and even Mollie the dog. I love sharing our planet together. Thanks, too, to my folks Arthur and Karla Lutz, my friends Saill and Alonza, and my other dear, dear friends, especially my best bud Tilly (who provided solitude, two ears, turkey meatloaf and low-fat brownies). For expertise, I thank Lisa Lewis, San Francisco fitness instructor and certified personal trainer; Jo Ann Hattner, Stanford University nutritionist; and Eric Thompson, manager of Omni Fitness Equipment Specialists in Oakland, California. On the publishing end, Andree Abecassis and Randy Ladenheim-Gil. Finally, I need to thank all the many teens whose insights I stole and wrote down, with extra special thanks to Hannah Margulis-Kessel, Josh Olsen, and Arden and Kim Bullard. And life wouldn't be complete without the Writergrrls.

Trademarks

All terms mentioned in this book that are known to be or are suspected of being trademarks or service marks have been appropriately capitalized. Alpha Books and Macmillan USA, Inc., cannot attest to the accuracy of this information. Use of a term in this book should not be regarded as affecting the validity of any trademark or service mark.

Part 1

Working Toward *Your* Ideal Body and Look

It's the beginning of something big! You want to look great; that's why you're reading this book. In the first part of the book, we'll talk about life as a teen, with a body that's sprouting and a mind that's expanding.

In this section, I'll give you some tools to start answering four big questions:

- ✦ *What do you really look like?*
- ✦ *What do you want to look like?*
- ✦ *How do you get there?*
- ✦ *What's getting in your way?*

You'll get suggestions, exercises, and a step-by-step approach to reaching your goals.

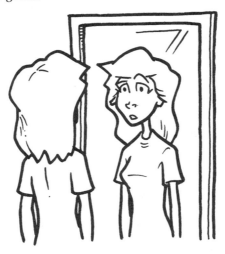

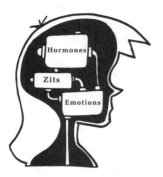

Chapter 1

Your Life in the Teen Machine

In This Chapter

✧ Chop, whirr, whizz ... you're in a change machine!

✧ The mind-body connection

✧ What's your self-image?

✧ A quick history of body fashions

✧ Thinking positive—and making the commitment to change

Psst! Come here! Wanna look great? Well, of course you do. Sit down here next to me; I'll let you in on some secrets. But before I do, I need to give you a warning: This is not a feel-good book that tells you how great you are, and how you should just accept what you look like because everybody is terrific just as they are. That feel-good stuff might be good for little kids and certain spacey grownups I've known, but it doesn't work for you. I mean, face it, you wouldn't have picked up this book unless you wanted to make a change or two in your life.

In this chapter we'll look at the connection between your mind and body. Since real change comes from within, you gotta have some self-knowledge to make those changes. And since this is the first chapter in the book, it makes sense to start at the beginning—where you are now. You'll be asking yourself some pretty important questions. So read through this chapter and the next (which is about where you want to be). Then the hard-core specifics of the rest of the book will make some real sense.

Life Inside the Teen Machine

You become a teen at 12, and it's like stepping into a giant change machine. Things whir, click, buzz, cut, saw, transmogrify, morph, and then ... eight years later, you step out again; voilà, you're a grown-up!

Whew. Wish it was so easy, or so mechanical.

Somehow, while you're in this "teen machine," your brain feels as scrambled as your body. You want to feel great and look great, but things are so confusing, life is moving so fast, and the stress is incredibly intense. Life is awesome and exciting, life is one big sorrowful drag. Your body changes, your friends change, your relationship with your parents changes ... a *lot*. Of course, there are school pressures, and the big question of what to do with your life. Relationships come and go. Zits happen. Hips and hair happen. Sometimes you just want to curl up in a ball and have your mom bring you a cup of hot chocolate.

Music helps. Friends help. Great activities help. Love helps. And working toward goals helps, too. Understanding yourself—who you are and what you want out of life—helps most of all.

The Body–Mind Connection

Your body and your mind are connected. Your thoughts, your behaviors, and your feelings all directly affect your health. It's all tied together:

✧ If you feed your body well, your mind will feel clear, active, and balanced.

✧ If your body is fit, your body will look great. You will enjoy the feeling, so you will feel great.

✧ If you feel great, you'll look great. If you look great, you'll feel great.

Let's look at where you are now: You're a teenager, and you want to look great. What's it like to be a teen? What are some of the influences on how you look—and how you feel about how you look? What do you think are some of the reasons you might look and feel the way you do?

PHAT Fact

If you're lost, a map to your destination won't do much good. You gotta know where you are—how you think and feel about your health and looks—before you choose which direction to travel.

Who and Where Are You Now?

Let's start with the here and now, the total basic facts.

If you're reading this book, you're probably a teen. That means you're between 12 and 20. I don't know anything else about you—your sex, your height, weight, interests, skills .... I don't know how much money your family has and whether or not that matters to you. I don't know what you dream about, or what language you speak at home with your parents. I don't know if you live with your parents. I don't know where you live, in what state, city, town ... in a house, apartment, group home, space port, homeless shelter, mansion, hotel, graveyard ... you get the picture.

I don't know anything about you ... but you do. And in this first chapter, I'd like you to focus on who you are. Because really looking at yourself—inside and out—is probably the most important part of making changes in yourself.

A Realistic View of You

A few years ago you were a kid. You might not have thought much about how you looked—many kids don't. That was before the hormones hit, and before your body started going wacky and wild, and sprouting in bizarre places. Now you look in the mirror and it's hard to know exactly how you look.

Some days, you're totally hot. Some days, you're not. Maybe it has to do with that pimple sprouting right on the tip of your nose. Maybe it has to do with the way your incredibly cute crush winked at you near your locker yesterday at school. Maybe it just has to do with the fact that you're seeing the world from a foot higher than you were last September.

PHAT Fact

The average female model is 5' 9$^1/_2$" inches and weighs 123 pounds. The average American woman is 5'4" tall and weighs 144 pounds.

Who you are and what you feel affects how you look. And that's not just your perception; all of that self-image, confidence, and health (or the lack of it) is mirrored on your face, in the dullness or shine of your hair and eyes, in your slumping, depressed posture or your strong, confident stride.

The Self-Suss Up

Okay. Pop quiz! It's time to assess where you are right now, because checking out how you feel about your looks is the first step to making changes. Take a few minutes … grab a pencil.

Write down your answers fast—you don't need to agonize over this. Usually the first thing that comes into your mind is the best. And don't worry about being wrong or stupid. In this pop quiz, the only wrong or stupid answers are the ones you don't write down. Ready? Begin.

What's your favorite part of your body?

What's your least favorite part?

What's interesting about your looks?

What's boring or ordinary about your looks?

What parts of you are beautiful?

Are you overweight, normal weight, or underweight?

How do you feel about your weight?

Have you ever been on a diet?

Do your friends and family like how you look? If they are critical of you, write a few ways how.

Do you look better clothed or undressed?

What do you think about the clothes you own? The clothes you wear?

What do you think about your skin?

Do you eat healthfully?

Do you want to know more about health and nutrition?

Are you physically fit?

What's your strongest physical skill?

What's your favorite exercise method or sport?

Write two things you like about your hair.

Write two things you don't like about your hair.

What's your style/look?

Now—quickly—list three things about your looks that you would like to improve.

Great! That's it! No, I'm not going to score this quiz, and neither are you. It's only intended to get you thinking about—and clarifying—your own opinions about *you.*

Your Sufferin' Self-Image!

A lot of times we don't have an accurate sense of what we look like. You might be looking too closely in the mirror at your body, or judging your actions, talents, skills, and qualities too harshly. You might look in the mirror and see a scrawny kid. You might look in the mirror and see nothing but big, fat hips, or the largest Adams apple in the world. But what you see in the mirror might have little to do with the reality of what you look like.

Sometimes self-image and body image get severely warped, and you might end up with an eating disorder. (There's a lot more about eating disorders in Chapter 7, "Help and Maintenance.")

Sometimes, even if you can really see what you do look like, you don't like what you see. You might torture yourself over your looks. Yep, a big part of being a teen is self-torture. You know, you really don't need to be so hard on yourself!

What Makes You Attractive?

Are you gorgeous? Are you a babe, a hottie, a hunk, a skank? Most of us don't feel like we look that great all the time. Part of that is what we see reflected in the world around us— billboards, magazines, TV shows. Of course, it's fairly bogus; even models don't look like models. Blame that perfect skin and thighs on that master of illusion: the photo retoucher and digital artist. With the right technology, you can shrink or enhance heads, smooth wrinkled skin, remove blemishes and zits, insta-lipo-suck fat away, and change eye colors. Real life never looks like that.

Even when you understand—really grasp—that people don't, won't, can't look perfect, it's hard to get your expectations of how you *should* look in line with how you *can* look, but it's a really good idea to work on getting these two things to balance.

So how do you figure out what you really look like? How attractive you really are? Guess what—it doesn't matter! If you change your emphasis from looking great to feeling great, you *will* look great. Promise. If you can forget about looking perfect and enjoy looking the best that you can, you'll avoid a lot of misery.

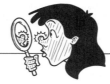

Beautiful? NOT!

Don't expect total clarity about what you want and need. Understanding yourself is tough because your body keeps changing, and new raging hormones keep messing with your mind.

It's Tough Being a Guy

Guys have tremendous pressures on them about body image. For them, there's a really narrow parameter of what looks great. If you're too short, too thin, too fat, too "feminine," you're probably gonna have a hard time. If you develop slower than the other guys. If your voice stays high. If you get pubic hair earlier than the other guys—or if you get it later. In some communities, if you don't like to fight. In other communities, if you aren't interested in—or good at— sports.

Some things you can change, and some you can't. But it's better to use your dissatisfaction with how you look as an incentive to change the things you can. You can always be healthier, stronger, more fit, better groomed. You can always feel better about yourself.

Bogus Beauty Standards for Women

Ninety-five percent of all girls and women don't look like models. You might waste endless hours and energy trying to get those big breasts, long legs, flat belly, and small hips—it won't work. You can only look like you—a fit version, to be sure—but you.

It's painful to be disappointed by your body. It's helpful to think about why we like certain body shapes. So much of it is based on *when* we're living in history.

Here's a quick 'n' dirty summary of some of the styles of the last 100 years or so.

The 1910s

Squish it and squash it, the corset was in! The idea was an hourglass figure, no matter what it did to women's internal organs (and boy, did it do it bad). What women did to get that waistline led to real physical trouble—not to mention how hard it is to breathe when your stomach is in your lungs.

The 1920s

The flapper was it, girl, and women bound their breasts to get a boyish profile. If you were busty, you were S.O.L.—no way you were gonna look great in those long, straight outfits.

PHAT Fact

My gorgeous Grandma Dolly, the one with the dimples and baby blue eyes, the great dancer, tortured herself all her life because of her large breasts. Her era was the '20s, when women were supposed to be flat as a boy.

The Late 1930s, Early 1940s

War time, the guys were off fighting, and women stepped into the work force to fill in the gap. That meant muscles, baby; a wiry, strong, look.

The 1950s

That curvy, bosomy look was where it was at, when the guys came back from war and women became housewives. Think of Marilyn Monroe. She'd be considered fat now. Was she fat then? No way! More like incredibly hot and sexy. If you were boyish in the 1950s, you would have agonized over boobs—and probably stuffed your pointy bra.

The 1960s

Twiggy (a model who looked like a twig) ruled. That meant straight lines (in hair and body). Breasts were out again. (Poor breasts, in, out, in, out ...)

The 1970s

Long and lean with big hair. Farrah hair. Think sex kitten with a gun. Oh, and a tan. All those hours in the sun, getting skin cancer, what a blast!

He Sez

"I didn't used to get Marilyn Monroe. I mean, she was kinda chunky, really. Then I saw this old movie. Man! She was awesome."

—Bill, age 19

The 1980s

Long and lean and muscular and taut. Not an ounce of fat on that toned bod. For girls and women who naturally have padding on breast, belly, and thigh, that's a hard (if not impossible) ideal to achieve. Ah … did we long for the 1950s! (Or the 1920s, 1930s, 1940s …)

The 1990s

Breast implants, liposuction, body sculpting; the perfect bod is within reach—if you've got the basic structure, the big bucks for surgery, and the willingness to change your body for an exterior image of how you should look.

And Now, and Soon?

What's the expectation? What kind of body do you wish you had? What's influencing your choice? What will they come up with next? (I sure hope it involves having a big butt.)

It's a Cultural Thing

Cultural standards of beauty also differ depending upon where you live. How you feel about your looks and body also depends on your culture. If you live in a part of the world where all the sexy people tend to be kinda large and you're thin and (maybe in your mind) just a bit scrawny, you're not gonna feel all that attractive, are you? If you're a blond and all the hot dudes have dark hair and skin, you might feel just a little bit out of it.

Size and beauty are more related in some cultures. In mainstream American culture, thinness seems to be vital. In some of the South Sea Island cultures, big *is* beautiful. The African-American culture tends to enjoy bigger women than the Caucasian-American culture does.

She Sez

"Most girls don't really care about what the models look like. Usually the media image is a petite girl with clear skin and perfect body and perfect face, but nobody is really like that."

—Kim, age 13

Becoming Who You Want to Be

It's hard to know how you want to look, how you want to be, and what you want to do when things are changing as fast as they are in the teen years. When I look at the historical breakdown I just gave you, and when I think about all these different ideas of beauty all over the world, I hear questions in my head:

✧ Doesn't it make you mad that each time in history has such a rigid idea about what makes a woman beautiful?

✧ Doesn't it seem sorta random?

✧ Isn't it a drag that you might be considered beautiful in one country but a "hag" here, or the reverse?

It takes internal strength to go against societal standards of beauty, whether they're based on time in history, or culture. It takes self-knowledge and self-confidence. It's hard work.

Totally Clueless?

Part of being a teen is that terrible feeling that you know nothing, and everybody knows more than you. Guess what? Nobody has a clue. That's why this book is full of specifics, like how to shave your legs, take your pulse during exercise, and wash your face. If nobody tells you how to become who you want to be, you're gonna farb around clueless for a long time. And that "clueless" feeling doesn't feel good.

When You Feel Ugly

It's common to hate some parts of you; it's far too normal to be completely self-critical. You hate your hair because it's not curly (your sister is dying for your long, smooth locks). You hate your beady little eyes and hawk nose (even though nobody sees them that way but you), and your skin! You just stare in the mirror and hate it! (Guess what, honey; from an inch away, everybody's skin is a disaster.) Stand back ... way back. Here's where the power of positive thinking comes in. In the next chapter, you'll learn about the "Looking Great" Journal and exercises to do (check out "The 'What's Wrong About My Body/What's Strong About My Body' Exercise" in Chapter 2). These are tools you can use when you're feeling bad about your looks.

It's Baby Steps, Baby!

There's no magic chill pill I can give you to make you feel groovy and gorgeous, centered, and stress-free. It's a process. I'm giving you a few tools—about eating, about exercise, and about beauty, but remember that change comes through taking baby steps—you can't figure it all out at once, and you can't change it all at once. The first baby step is trusting that you can make changes in your life.

If you're having a hopeless moment (we all have them ...) try these techniques:

✧ Think positive. Force yourself. Choose what you want, and act as if it's a done deal. Tell yourself again and again, "I'm gonna look great by next month!" When you feel hopeless, play a little game with yourself. Pretend that you're full of hope. Pretend that you already *know* you can change yourself.

✧ Make the commitment to change. If you decide to change yourself—really make that decision—then you'll have made a commitment to yourself. It's like a marriage commitment. You're promising to stick with yourself in sickness and in health, for richer or for poorer.

✧ Use your "Looking Great" Journal (in Chapter 2) to notice how you feel. Looking at monsters usually makes them disappear.

The Least You Need to Know

✧ The teen years are about change—to your body, mind, relationships, and ideas. No wonder you feel uneven.

✧ How you look *is* directly related to how you feel—and the reverse.

✧ Checking out how you feel about your looks is the first step to making changes.

✧ Forget about looking perfect; enjoy looking the best that you can, and you'll avoid a lot of misery.

✧ Body styles change throughout history. What's pretty now might be horrendous in a few years.

✧ It's normal to feel ugly sometimes.

✧ You *can* make changes in your looks and your life.

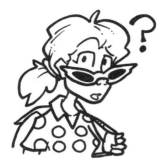

Chapter 2

Improvement!? You're Not Out to Lunch

In This Chapter

✧ Four steps to making change

✧ Groovin' with your goals

✧ Taking tiny steps (and lots of them)

✧ Getting around the "uglies" on your way to making change

✧ Exercises for your "Looking Great" Journal

Hey, you're a realist. You don't look as great as you want to, but you're smart about it—you know you're not going to look like your favorite MTV VJ or supermodel (they have a lot of professional staff working on their images—and they don't even look as great as you think they do). You also know you've got room for improvement. And you do want to look better. You want to look great!

As you'll find out in later chapters, looking great comes primarily from being healthy and fit. The other stuff—hair, nails, fashion, and all that—comes afterward. Don't worry, we'll get to all of it in a few pages.

This chapter focuses on helping you to set realistic goals and meet them. Staying motivated is always easier once you start meeting goals, so it's important to set goals you can meet—and set up the steps you'll need to take to get there. Then it's just like paint-by-numbers. Break it down into doable pieces, and then do the pieces.

Yeah, right. I know, it's not so easy as all that. So I'll give you a few tools and tips to help.

Change, Change, Got Spare Change?

Getting from A to Z is a long journey, and you don't want to get stuck somewhere in the L-M-N-O-P part. So I've broken the process of making changes in your looks (or life) into four steps. Making changes means

1. Deciding what goals you want to achieve.

2. Figuring out the right steps to take to get there.

3. Taking—slowly and deliberately—those right steps.

4. Celebrating your success—at every step of the process.

It sounds so easy when broken down like that. But each of these four steps can be difficult. In the rest of the chapter we'll look at these steps a little closer.

Step One: Setting Your "Looking Great" Goals

Let's talk about goals. A goal is something you aim for in life. In a ball game like soccer, a goal is a fairly small area of the playing field where you try to get the ball. In basketball, it's a hoop. It's not a vague "oh, somewhere over there ..."; it's specific. And any goals you make regarding your looks should be specific, too. Saying, "Yeah man, I wanna look so cool that every hottie in the place will fall down moaning" is not a specific goal. There's no way to reach that goal, because there's nowhere to start.

Not Just What, But When

When you set a specific goal, make sure to include the time-line. Think of a long-term goal as something you want to happen within the next few months, or the next year.

For instance, I might decide my goals are to ...

Run five miles a day by May.

or ...

Blast 'em in a bikini by next June.

The timeline can seem kinda random. That's okay for now. A goal is somewhere—and somewhen—to aim your efforts.

Introducing: Your "Looking Great" Journal!

How will you set these goals and establish the timelines? You can start doing it here, in this book, but it's much better if you build yourself a "Looking Great" Journal. It's totally easy; here's how:

✧ Get a notebook.

✧ Find a pen you love.

✧ Write "Looking Great!" on the outside of the notebook (or not, if that seems too dumb).

✧ Meet your new friend, your "Looking Great" Journal.

But ... Why?

Moving through this book is about setting goals and reaching them, and it's hard to do that without keeping a record. Your "Looking Great" Journal is not a diary (that little book with the lock you got for your eighth birthday and never really wrote in after the second week). Even if you're not really into writing, a journal can be really helpful—both at the time you're writing in it, 'cause it gives you a way to express your emotions, and later on, to get a sense of your progress.

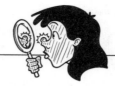

Beautiful? NOT!

Hey, this is not an all-purpose notebook. Dedicate your "Looking Great" Journal to this one purpose. No math problems in the back, no notes to your friends in the middle.

What Do You Write About?

This journal is ...

- ✧ For learning more about yourself.
- ✧ For setting goals and timelines.
- ✧ For planning the steps to meet those goals.
- ✧ For having a place to vent.
- ✧ For noticing things about yourself, your body, and the world.
- ✧ For keeping a record of your progress.

If you keep a journal ...

- ✧ You won't forget where you started from.
- ✧ You'll be able to figure out what works—and what doesn't work—for you.

There are "Looking Great" Journal exercises sprinkled through this chapter. I've put a bunch of them at the end of the chapter, too.

Setting Your Long-Term Goals Exercise

Why not start with establishing your long-term goals?

Write in your journal (or here): I want to ____do what____ by
____when____ .

I want to _____ by _____.

Got several goals?

I want to _____ by _____.

I want to _____ by _____.

Hold on, not too many now! You don't want to set yourself
up to be overwhelmed. (If you're having trouble figuring out
what goals to choose, why not do "The Nailing Down Your
Goals Exercise" at the end of this chapter? Feeling any clearer
now?)

PHAT Fact

Reaching your goals means staying aware that you want to
make changes, clearly identifying what they are, and making daily (sometimes hourly) choices to move toward those
changes.

Doing Step 2. How Do I Get There?

To achieve your long-term goals, you need short-term goals.
Short-term goals are your stepping stones on the way, because goals don't just happen. Your short-term goals are your
strategies. (If you're the kind of person who lives for the moment, it might be hard to set these—but it's really important
to try.) Here are some tips:

✧ Keep short-term goals as action steps; things you will *do* rather than things you will *be*. For example, "This week, I'll eat dessert after dinner instead of before lunch" is an action step. Yes! That's the kind of short-term goal that's framed as an action. "I'll be more disciplined about eating sweets" isn't. It won't work. It's too vague.

✧ Make your short-term goals very short-term. "I will take a walk today after school" instead of "I'm gonna walk twice a week for the next six months."

✧ Make your short-term goals doable. Be realistic. Don't bite off more than you can easily chew.

Say, for instance, that your goal is to run five miles a day by May. Once you read Chapter 10, "Outside Exercise and Team Sports," you'll have a better idea of how to start. (Hint: Start by walking, and start by getting good shoes.) Your short-term goals would include:

1. Read Chapter 10 by Friday.

2. Get Mom to take me shoe shopping Tuesday. (You might have an interim step—earn shoe money by baby-sitting, for instance).

3. Start by walking two miles a day, three times a week for the next two weeks, beginning Wednesday.

4. ... and so on.

PHAT Fact

Goals should always include a time element.

Exercise: Your Short-Term Goals

Get out your journal. At the top of a blank page, write one of your long-term goals (don't forget to write the "by when" part). Now here's the hard part: figuring out the steps you need to take to meet your goals. This is something you're going to come back to—after you read the parts of this book that apply!

List the specific steps you're gonna take.

1. _____
2. _____
3. _____
4. _____

... and so on.

She Sez

"I get freaked out when I think about how much weight I have to lose. I think it's better to just think about eating healthy today. It's not so overwhelming."

—Sara, age 16

Step 3. Taking the Right Steps

If you have your short-term goals in mind, you don't need to be overwhelmed by long-term goals. Whew! Just concentrate on the small pieces of meeting the little goals.

And that means making choices, sometimes every day, sometimes every hour! You have a lot of opportunities for success. Let's say you're a junk food junkie and you hate how you feel.

You want to improve your energy level, and after reading this book, you've come back to this chapter to nail down your goals. You've decided that your long-term goal is to get healthier by eating whole foods, and you've decided that Thanksgiving is your long-term target date (let's say it's about six months away). You've decided that, as a step to getting off the junk food, you'll make healthier choices at the school cafeteria where you buy your lunch. Your short-term goal is to eat fruit instead of chips at lunchtime for the next three weeks.

Easy enough. Now it's lunch time. You're hungry, it's a lousy day, and you're bummed that your crush likes your best friend instead of you, so you head for the chips. STOP! Make the choice to get an apple, instead. It's a little thing—yet it's a big step on the way to getting off the junk food.

The great thing about such small goals is that you don't even need to make the right choice every time! If you meet your small goals 75 percent of the time, that's great. Because, after all, nobody is perfect, and nobody is 100 percent consistent. (We'd be boring automatons if we were.) Think about it: Tomorrow arrives, and soon it's lunch time. There you are in the lunch line, grabbing for the chips. Wait! You can make the choice again, right here. Put those chips back. There's a juicy orange waiting for you at the end of the line ....

PHAT Fact

It's not easy identifying your long-term goals. That might be the hardest part of the process. If you're not sure what your goal should be, try picking one, any healthy one, at random. Work toward it. Your real needs and goals will probably emerge.

Step 4. Cool! Celebrating Your Success

Okay, now I'm gonna lecture. It's really, really, really important to let yourself celebrate your successes. That might mean giving yourself a high five whenever you choose apples over chips, and it might mean buying yourself a new CD when you pass your first martial arts test and turn in your white belt for a colored one. Giving yourself credit for your accomplishments is part of the "looking great" credo.

Ugly Things in the Way

It's important not to punish yourself for not achieving your goals. You might have set them too high, or messed up on the timeline. It's more important to keep working toward what you want. It can be hard to convince yourself of that, though, especially when the Uglies start crawling out from under the rug to tease you and make you feel bad.

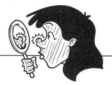

Beautiful? NOT!

Don't let the Uglies get you down! Try writing about them in your "Looking Great" Journal. Uglies usually disappear when examined closely.

Uglies are things you tell yourself that get in the way between you and your goals. Uglies—like all monsters—usually go away when they're looked at.

The Time Ugly—"But My Date's Next Week!"

The Time Ugly—truly a terrible monster—attacks your patience. I know, you want to lose weight, and you want to lose weight *now*. Your skin is a disaster, what are you gonna do about that zit on your nose? The Time Ugly comes out when you hang your self-esteem on reaching your goal, when you feel so bad about yourself that you have no patience for change—you need to feel better immediately (of course!) so you want the change to happen immediately.

The Time Ugly's message is painful. The answer, unfortunately, is that change just takes time. In the meantime, work on feeling better about yourself, no matter what you look like, and celebrating the fact that you're actually taking positive steps toward looking great. Celebrating the little achievements helps. Using the stress relief methods in Chapter 18, "Stress Busting," can help, too.

The Vanity Ugly—"She Can't See Me Like This!"

When you're feeling bad about yourself—on the inside—it's too easy to push that feeling onto the outside.

I remember traveling halfway across the country, in a city where my old friend Mikelle was living, and unable to pick up the phone to call her. My excuse to myself? I was 5 or 10 pounds heavier than I was when I last saw her—over 10 years ago. Now I'm the first one to admit that that kind of thinking is pathetic.

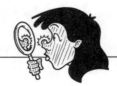

Beautiful? NOT!

Nobody cares about your looks like you do. Don't use your oh-so-normal flaws to keep you from experiencing life.

The point is, the main person—really the only person—concerned about and obsessed about your weight or your zits is you. Missing an event, or even feeling bad about it, because of a few pounds or pimples is tragic. Leave it behind you, do the best you can, and have fun anyway.

The Frantic Ugly—"But I'm Too Busy!"

Of course you're busy, and of course it's impossible to work big change into your schedule. That's why you make your short-term goals small. When the Frantic Ugly starts whispering nasty little messages in your ear, have it read the section on short-term goals (do Step 2, "How Do I Get There?").

The Misunderstood Ugly—"Everybody Else Is Being a Jerk!"

Sometimes Uglies tell the truth; sometimes everybody else is being a jerk. When you change, it makes your friends think about themselves in a new way. The same goes for your family. When you make changes in your eating, for instance, your parents might feel that they're being rejected—after all, they fed you a certain way all your life. It helps to have the support of people who believe in you and believe in the changes you're trying to make.

Whatever area of your health, nutrition, exercise, or appearance you're trying to improve, you can find people to support you—if you only look. Here are several ideas for building your "Looking Great" Support Team:

✧ **Your parents.** I know, I just said they might feel rejected. They might also feel really pleased that you're trying to make improvements. Ask for their help, and incorporate them into reaching your goals. There's more on this in Chapter 5, "Changes and Choices in Food."

✧ **Your current friends.** If you have friends that want to set—and meet—goals with you, you'll all have a better time doing it! Share this book with them. Maybe you want to exercise together, watch your weight together, or give each other home facials.

✧ **Therapists and counselors.** Sometimes you need to pull in the big guns. There's more on this in Chapters 7, "Help and Maintenance," and 18.

✧ **New friends.** If you're doing new activities, you're likely to meet new people who are interested in the same things you are. They can be a big support, too.

The Rigid Ugly—"That's Not What You Said You Would Do!"

Goals are something to aim toward. So you can't run five miles because you learn that your knees are weak, and running isn't possible ... or you end up on the swim team (that's where all your buds are, anyway) so you never have time to run. Or, you've grown two inches and kept the same weight, so you feel slimmer, but come June, you still prefer how you look in a one-piece Speedo instead of that bikini you've been eyeing. Are you a failure because you didn't exactly meet your goals? No, you are not. You are a success. You've improved, and you're looking great—you were flexible, and flexible isn't copping out. Here are two mottoes that might feel useful:

- ✧ Don't Marry the Goal
- ✧ Get flexible!

The Failure Ugly—"You've Blown It, Baby!"

You didn't walk even once this week, and your short-term goal was to walk three times. Oh, there were reasons. First, Uncle Pete came to town and you had to go with your brother to pick him up at the airport. Then, you had a test in chemistry, and you had to study. Then ... whatever. It didn't happen.

Now, since you've blown it, you wanna just ditch it. You feel so bad about yourself that you're chucking the whole thing. Don't! Fergeddaboutit. Start again. Think about your short-term goal, to walk three times a week. Maybe it's just not possible with your schedule. Maybe you need to take another step in between to build in time. Go back to the long-term goal list and look at what you want. Break it down again into little steps. Short-term goals are flexible. There are a lot of ways to get the ball down the court and to the basket.

He Sez

"I used to set goals at school, but I wasn't really motivated to follow them. Unless you really believe in them, it's not going to work."

—Jordan, age 19

Self-Respect, Moderation, and Loving Your Body

Okay, here's another big secret—taking care of your body is deeply satisfying. You might think you're giving up a lot—you're not. Taking care of yourself doesn't mean sacrificing—anything. Nothing in this book urges you to go for extreme behavior (starving yourself, avoiding all junk food, or giving up anything you love doing). It's a moderate approach.

By eating more moderately, taking time to exercise, and caring for your looks, you're simply being respectful and loving of yourself. You're making healthy changes so you can look great from the inside out. When you act respectfully to yourself, it's not really so grim, is it? It's the opposite of grim. It feels great. It's fun. It's an adventure with—and for—yourself.

More "Looking Great" Journal Exercises

You can use your "Looking Great" journal simply to define your goals and keep track of your progress, and you can use it to vent. You can also use it to learn a little more about yourself—your wants, your needs, your feelings about yourself. Here are some exercises to try. How about one every day, or for the busy, one a week?

29

The Nailing Down Your Goals Exercise

Spend a few minutes answering each of the following four questions. Be sure to be specific.

1. What do I look like now?
2. How do I want to look?
3. What do I want to change in my life?
4. By when do I want this change to happen?

The "Three Things That Went Okay Today, Three Things That Sucked" Exercise

This exercise is good to do every day—it keeps you in touch with what's going on outside your head. This helps keep you balanced (for example, you realize, "No, I'm not losing my mind, I'm simply under a lot of stress because of the car accident and the bad news about Grandpa!")

Went okay:

1. _____
2. _____
3. _____

Sucked:

1. _____
2. _____
3. _____

The "What's Wrong About My Body?/What's Strong About My Body?" Exercise

How do you really feel about your looks? Try doing this exercise, and then do it again a few weeks later. It's usually interesting to see the differences.

Quick. Write down the first three things you think of when asked, "What's wrong about your body?

1. _____

2. _____

3. _____

Now, write down the first three things you think of when asked, "What's strong about your body?"

1. _____

2. _____

3. _____

I've heard it said that the longest journey begins with a single step. Whoever said that was one wise dude or dudess. It's true! You can't get anywhere unless you begin. These first two chapters were your beginning. Now it's time to move on to the journey. Got your bags packed and your shoes on? Let's do it.

She Sez

"My favorite thing on me is my eyes; they're green and they're pretty bright. I like those. I don't like my nose because it looks round on the front but it's pointy from the side view. It's pretty weird."

—Kim, age 13

The Least You Need to Know

✧ Make your long-term goals specific, and include a time-line.

✧ Short-term goals are your strategies. Keep them doable!

✧ Your "Looking Great" Journal gives you a way to express your emotions and a sense of your progress.

✧ You reach your goals by making small choices every day.

✧ If you do 75 percent of your short-term goals, you're doing great. Nobody's perfect!

✧ Celebrate your successes, large and small!

✧ Don't let the uglies get you down. Take a good look at them and watch them fade away.

✧ Shhh! Don't tell! Taking care of your body is deeply sat-isfying.

Part 2

Healthy Eating

Food—it's the gas for your car, the tiger in your tank, the staff (and stuff) of life. You gotta eat to live (and some of us live to eat!)

This section is all about food: thinking about it, understanding it, shopping for it, cooking it and … oh yeah … eating it. You'll learn about what we mean by "healthy" food, what food contains what nutrients, and the scoop on organics, vegetarianism, and when to eat what for your health, for getting to sleep, and for staying energetic. Eating well is key to looking—and feeling—great. And that's what you're reading this for, right?

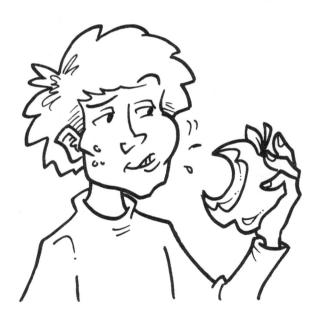

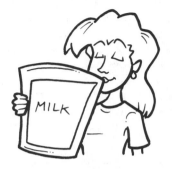

Chapter 3

Balanced Diet 101— Teen Style

In This Chapter

✧ The basics of balancing what you eat

✧ The inside scoop on what teens need in their diet

✧ Understanding the Food Guide Pyramid

✧ More tips for eating the good stuff

You know that saying, "Garbage in, garbage out"? As a teen, your body's got some specific needs. In order to look great and feel your best, you've got to eat the right things. Nutrition is a simple matter of input and output—when you put good food in, you get good looks and energy out.

This is a detail chapter—in this chapter we'll look at the nuts and breads (I mean nuts and bolts) of your specific nutritional needs. (By the way, you'll notice that I'm not talking about prepared foods such as hamburgers, Thai noodle salad, or Chicken Caccitore. No, this chapter is about ingredients, nutrients, and serving sizes. We'll put them together later on.)

Making Healthy Food = Tasty Food

Food has got to taste good, and eating is—and should be—one of life's pleasures. If you just listen to your old health teacher droning on about vitamins and minerals, you might feel like you're gonna end up like some sort of 1960s weirdo, eating nothing but dry and tasteless whole grains and sea-weed (kombu, anyone?). That's not true. Healthy food can be the tastiest and most fun of all. Think fresh. Fresh fruit. Chicken grilled on the barbecue dripping with natural juices. Vegetables that aren't over-cooked. Food prepared so you can taste the flavors ... yum!

Of course, food is a matter of taste and habit. But even if you're totally hooked on Pringles and your idea of health food is cotton-candy flavor Go-gurt ("It's yogurt, right?" ... "Well, yogurt-*based*"), you can still make some positive and healthy changes.

PHAT Fact

Eating well is key to long-lasting health. Good nutrition re-sults from eating the foods in the right quantities, with the right nutrients, over the long term.

... and don't stress too much about balancing every meal. Focus on balancing your eating patterns over a few days. That means that, no, you haven't destroyed the entire good eating thing if you pig out on ice cream on the weekend. So long as most of the time you eat fairly low-fat, high-fiber foods: vegetables, fruits and whole grains (and you don't eat too much or too little of them), you'll be eating well.

Stuff *Your* Bod Needs to Be Healthy

Your body is growing rapidly, and puberty puts special strains on it. Because you're growing so fast, you've got to eat a lot. You've got specific dietary needs that kids and full-grown adults don't have.

You've also got some eating "challenges" based on two facts: Most teens eat away from home more often (which means it's harder to regulate what you eat), and most teens eat a lot of fast food (which is very yummy but not all that nutritious). The fact is, most teens don't get anywhere near their nutritional requirements. That means that—right there— you're not going to look and feel your best.

How can you fix or enhance your eating habits? Before you figure out what you should be eating (and how you should eat it), you gotta know what you need.

She Sez

"Maybe I'm weird, but I really like lentils and beans and brown rice and stuff like that. I can feel the nutrition just flowing into my body."

—Alyssa, age 15

Increase the Iron

As a male teen, you need about 20 percent more iron than you did as a preadolescent. As a female teen, you need about 33 percent more iron—especially once you begin your period. (Menstruation drains iron from your body, so it's important to replace it with an iron-rich diet.) Iron is found in red meats as well as in a number of vegetables and grains. Some of the top iron-containing foods are tofu (a mild smooth and dense soy bean product that's the basis of a lot of vegetarian cooking), cream of wheat, dried fruits, Swiss chard and other dark, leafy greens, artichokes, tomato paste, lentils, beans, beet greens, chick peas, and pumpkin.

Count on Calcium—Your Bones Do!

Your bones are growing rapidly. Eat foods that help—rather than interfere with—bone growth! Fifteen percent of your height is added during your teen years, and calcium is an essential ingredient for boosting those bones. You need about 1,200 milligrams of calcium a day. If you don't like—or can't tolerate—milk and milk products (always a great source of calcium), try tofu, spinach, artichokes, rhubarb, beet greens, kale, beans, chickpeas, pumpkin, and sweet potatoes. (Does this list sound familiar to you? A lot of foods that are high in iron are high in calcium, too.)

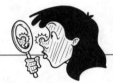

Beautiful? NOT!

Soft drinks contain phosphoric acid, which robs your body of calcium. Calcium is desperately needed for bone growth! When it comes to beverages, stick with water as much as you can—cool, clear, refreshing water!

Power Yourself with Protein

Especially for guys, protein needs go up—way up—in the teen years. Proteins are found in meats and also in beans of all kinds. Artichokes also have protein, as do broccoli, spinach, kale, peas, asparagus, and beet greens.

Slink with Zinc

What's zinc? Zinc is a mineral used by your immune system to help produce white blood cells. There is lots of zinc in artichokes, beans, and chickpeas.

Vitalize with Vitamins

As a teen, your daily needs for vitamins go up 20 to 30 percent. This might be a time to think about taking a daily multivitamin.

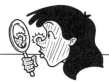

Beautiful? NOT!

Too much zinc can actually hurt your immune system function. Skip the supplements, and stick to getting your zinc from foods.

Wallow in Water

Water flushes your system, keeps things running, and clears your skin. Especially if you exercise, you need a lot of fluids—and that means water. (Juice—in limited quantities—is good, too. Soft drinks are considerably less good for you—plus they often contain caffeine, and too much caffeine leads to problems. Diet soft drinks are even worse—you're basically dumping a bunch of chemicals in your body—*not* healthy.)

I Know the Food Guide Pyramid Seems Boring, But ...

So what should you be eating? And how much of it? A number of years ago, the U.S. Department of Agriculture (USDA) developed the Food Guide Pyramid, which gives the suggested diet for health in an easy-to-understand graphic. Now, it's everywhere. You've probably seen it on classroom walls so often it's become wallpaper, covering up the cracks.

The Food Guide Pyramid may be boring, but because it shows people *visually* the healthiest way to eat, it's helped a lot of people improve their nutrition. Check it out again; it can be a helpful tool.

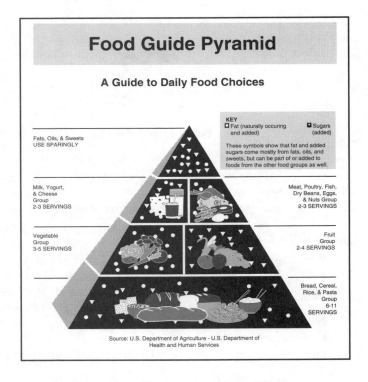

Food Guide Pyramid

A Guide to Daily Food Choices

KEY
☐ Fat (naturally occuring and added)   ◼ Sugars (added)

These symbols show that fat and added sugars come mostly from fats, oils, and sweets, but can be part of or added to foods from the other food groups as well.

Fats, Oils, & Sweets
USE SPARINGLY

Milk, Yogurt, & Cheese Group
2-3 SERVINGS

Meat, Poultry, Fish, Dry Beans, Eggs, & Nuts Group
2-3 SERVINGS

Vegetable Group
3-5 SERVINGS

Fruit Group
2-4 SERVINGS

Bread, Cereal, Rice, & Pasta Group
6-11 SERVINGS

Source: U.S. Department of Agriculture - U.S. Department of Health and Human Services

The Food Guide Pyramid breaks food into different groups: bread, cereal, rice, and pasta; vegetables; fruits; milk products; meats and other proteins; and fats, oils, and sweets. It gives a range of how much of each category you should eat to feel and look good.

The Food Guide Pyramid stresses that you need foods from each and every category to be healthy. You can't just eat vegetables, and you can't just eat sugar—and I'm not talking about long-term results—eating a mono-diet or a diet deficient in key nutrients will show up pretty fast in how you feel, look, and act (think oily skin and low energy).

Taking the Pyramid with a Grain of Salt

The Food Guide Pyramid is not perfect. It can help you with balance and quantity of food, but it says nothing about food quality. Nuts and beans (terrific, healthy foods) are in the same category as meat, for instance, even though they have very different effects on the body. Fats are all considered "bad" even though unsaturated oils like flaxseed, olive, and canola oils are high in Omega-3 acids, which are essential for health. And white bread is lumped with brown bread even though white bread has far less fiber—it's just not as healthy for you, plus it tastes kinda bland.

You'll also notice that the pyramid says nothing about calories or amounts of nutrients and fats. That's great as far as I'm concerned—using the pyramid as a guide to eating well takes the stress off of counting fat grams and calories and puts the stress back where it belongs, on eating to feel and look good.

PHAT Fact

The Food Guide Pyramid shows a range of suggested servings. Where do you fall? Here's a tip: A small, inactive woman would be at the bottom of the range; a big, athletic, teenage guy would be at the high end of the range.

Serves You Right!

The other confusing thing about the Food Guide Pyramid is: What the #$%^# do they mean by a "serving"? Don't get the idea that if you sit down to a plate of food, that plateful equals one serving. Then you're like, "Mom, can I have another serving?" and she slops another huge glob of whatever on your plate, and that's another serving .... Not so! So ... what does "serving" mean?

Great Grains Galore!

Bread, Cereal, Rice, and Pasta, these are the foundation of the pyramid. This is the food group that should make up most of your daily diet. The Food Guide Pyramid suggests 6 to 11 servings a day. That sounds like a lot, until you realize what they mean by a "serving." For the grain group, a serving is ...

- ✧ 1 ounce of ready-to-eat cereal (this is measured by weight, because so much boxed cereal contains so much air—think Rice Crispies). A lot of boxed cereals are "empty food" without much nutrition. Remember the rule of trying to eat close to the source.

- ✧ One slice of bread (which makes your lunch sandwich two servings, and the bread on each piece of pizza one serving—don't forget to count the cheese and pepperoni!). Whole-grain breads are healthier (and more satisfying) than that white fluff that passes for bread in some places—the high fiber is terrific for you. Go easy on the high-fat bread spreads, too (use mustard instead of mayo).

- ✧ $1/2$ cup of cooked cereal (like oatmeal), rice, or pasta. That plate of spaghetti Mom threw in front of you, then, is at least two servings, maybe three. Since whole grain is healthier, lean toward brown rice and whole-wheat or enriched pasta when possible.

Veritable Vegetables

Vegetables range from leafs to roots—humans, because we're omnivores who devour a bit of everything, eat all sorts of veggies, too, in all sorts of preparations. For vegetables, the pyramid suggests three to five servings a day and counts one serving as ...

- ✧ 1 cup of raw, leafy vegetables (salad fixings).
- ✧ $^1/_2$ cup of other vegetables either cooked or chopped raw (I'm thinking salsa here).

PHAT Fact

White is wrong; brown is better—at least when it comes to food. White rice and bread (and even white potatoes) have fewer nutrients in them than brown rice and bread (and darker potatoes such as yams).

- ✧ $^3/_4$ cup of vegetable juice (but really, just how much tomato and carrot juice can you drink before growing vegetables out of your nose?).

Freaky Fruit

In the summer, there's nothing better than fresh, juicy watermelon and sweet cherries; in the fall and winter, crisp apples, succulent pears ... Frozen and canned fruit is healthy, too. The Food Guide Pyramid recommends two to four servings of fruit a day, and one serving equals ...

- ✧ One medium apple, orange, banana (or nectarine, peach, two apricots, and so on).

- ❖ $^1/_2$ chopped, cooked, or canned fruit.
- ❖ $^3/_4$ cup of fruit juice (so that large glass of OJ in the morning gets you most of the way there).

PHAT Fact

Veggie crunch! It's hard to eat too many vegetables. Vegetables are high in nutrients and fiber and low in calories. Few Americans eat anywhere near the recommended servings of vegetables—and the recommendation only states the minimum!

Meaningful Milk, Yogurt, and Cheese

Milk products are especially meaningful for teens because of the teen need for increased calcium. The Food Guide Pyramid recommends at least two servings daily of nonfat or low-fat milk, yogurt, and cheese. I'd add at least one more for teens. So what do they mean by a "serving"?

- ❖ 1 cup of milk or yogurt
- ❖ $1^1/_2$ ounces of natural cheese (1 ounce of cheese is about the size of your thumb—unless you're the biggest klutz in the world—"all thumbs" … okay, I'll shut up)
- ❖ 2 ounces of processed cheese (though really, with all the incredible cheeses in the world, why bother with the processed stuff?)

Magnificent Meat, Poultry, Fish, Dry Beans, Eggs, and Nuts (Whew!)

The Food Guide Pyramid recommends two to three servings of these protein-heavy foods. For vegetarians (see Chapter 5), that means the beans, eggs, and nuts (tofu, because it is made from soybeans, is the vegetarian's delight, so it goes in this category, too). And a serving is (drumroll, please) …

❖ 2 to 3 ounces of cooked lean meat, poultry, or fish (Three ounces is about the size of a deck of cards. That means that a thick, juicy steak probably satisfies your meat needs for the day. You'll notice that they say "lean." Try your meat skinless, broiled, roasted, or simmered instead of breaded and fried.)

❖ $1/2$ cup of cooked dry beans or one egg is the same as one ounce of lean meat. One-third cup of nuts or 2 tablespoons of nut butter also counts as 1 ounce of lean meat. Beans are among the healthiest foods.

Sugars, Fats, Oils, and Other "Sinful" Substances

Some fats and sugars are a necessary part of your diet, but butter and margarine, oil, candy, high-fat salad dressing, and soft drinks add little. You don't need these things to satisfy your nutritional needs.

Hey, by the way, I'm not suggesting a lifestyle without any of these foods, or without *any* fats and sugars. Most people need some of these to feel fully satisfied in their diet and life …. Just try to keep processed sugars to under 10 percent of your diet, keep those saturated fats to 10 percent or less, and focus on eating healthfully most of the time. I'm a big believer in the slogan "Everything in moderation, including moderation." (Also see the snacking suggestions in Chapter 4.)

Digesting the Pyramid

The Food Guide Pyramid is not the only key to healthy nutrition. Yes, use it as a way to balance your eating. But also keep the following tips in mind.

Go for Variety

Eat a variety of foods (no mono-diets, where you only eat grapefruit [bleck!], mashed potatoes, or French toast for weeks on end). When it comes to food, variety truly is the spice of life! There is no one perfect food. You need a true combination to get the nutrients you need.

Moderate Your Meat

Eat your meat lean. Shift your emphasis from *meat* and potatoes to *potatoes* and meat. You don't need to eliminate meat from your diet, but it is healthy to emphasize the vegetables.

He Sez

"I love my meat but I love my fruits, too. Give me a nectarine, and I'm stoked."

—Danny, age 13

Don't Forget the Oil!

A number of vegetable oils have their place in a healthy diet (olive, flax, canola, soy)—about 1 tablespoon a day, ideally. These oils contain Omega-3 fatty acids, which make your eyes shine, your hair glow, and your skin radiate. They also help reduce the incidence of heart attacks in older people. Palm and coconut oils are not so good—they tend to be processed into hydrogenated oils to make them solid. Solid fats clog up the works in your body.

Try to reduce your saturated fat intake. No more than 30 percent of your total diet should come from fats (this includes "good" fats—the unsaturated kind found in vegetables, and "bad" fats—the saturated fats found mostly in animal products).

PHAT Fact

Trust your body. People are born knowing when they are hungry and when they are full. Unfortunately, we've learned to ignore our own internal signals. Listen to your hunger and fullness. Your body knows what it needs (right now my body is telling me it needs a massage and a trip to a tropical island in Thailand—how about yours?).

Ah, the Complexity of Carbohydrates ...

Choose a diet with lots of grains, veggies, and fruit. These are key because they have complex carbohydrates (starch and fiber), vitamins, and minerals. Few people—even dieters—get enough of these foods.

High Fiber Rules!

What's the fuss about fiber? Dietary fiber is found only in plants. Fiber comes in two types: insoluble fiber (also known as roughage) and soluble fiber. Insoluble fiber keeps things going in the digestive tract, if you know what I mean. The skins of fruits and vegetables, whole grains, wheat, and corn bran all are good sources of insoluble fiber. Soluble fiber helps reduce the risk of heart trouble and helps control blood sugar.

A Few More Short and Sweet Tips

Eating well can be complicated, but here are some more simple tips to help you on your way.

- ✧ **Be sensible with salt.** Be salt-moderate (this is *not* where to practice shakin' it). Try *not* salting your food.

Spices and pepper and a squeeze of fresh lemon often taste just as yummy, and make your body a lot happier.

✧ **Oh joy, it's soy!** Enjoy soy, a high-protein, high-calcium, and high-nutrient food. That means tofu, soy-milk, and those yummy Japanese soybeans, edamame!

✧ **Watch that sugar!** Desserts can be wonderful—if you keep them to two to three servings a week. Keep your overall sugar intake low. Keep candy, soda, and sweet drinks to a minimum.

✧ **Eat naturally.** Go for the less-processed foods. Pure food is where it's at. Avoid artificial coloring, hydro-genated oils, and nitrites.

✧ **Move your body.** Balance your food with physical ac-tivity (lots more on that later in the book).

The Least You Need to Know

✧ What you eat affects almost everything about you.

✧ Focus on balancing your food types and moderating your portions.

✧ Because you're growing so fast, teens have specific nutri-tional needs.

✧ The Food Guide Pyramid is helpful for selecting foods and balancing portions (but it doesn't help you deter-mine quality).

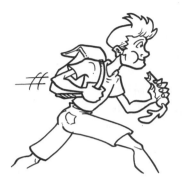

Chapter 4

Eating on the Run— Eating for Your Lifestyle

In This Chapter

✦ Your Basic Eating Plan—five steps to feeling great

✦ Breakfast basics, lunching logic, dinner do's

✦ Snack-a-doodle-doo! Snacks are good for you!

✦ Great healthy foods on-the-go

✦ What to eat to sleep

It's one thing to know what kinds of food are healthy to eat and the best proportions to eat them in. But how does that translate to daily life? Life is full enough with school, home, and other stuff. Who has time to plan healthy meals and then actually make sure that healthy food is around to eat?

Here's the thing: It may take a little reorganization now, but shortly you'll find that it's just as easy to make good, healthy food choices.

Your Basic Eating Plan

Ready for your Basic Eating Plan? It's pretty basic (that's why it's called the ... I know).

1. **Pay attention to what you eat.** Human beings eat a lot and eat frequently. Much of the time we're not really aware of what—or how much—we eat. A lot of people aren't even aware of what they like and don't like to eat! It's in front of us, we eat it. The first step to changing what you eat is to notice what you eat. (You don't need to write it down, just notice it.)

2. **Understand what makes a good, nutritious diet, and try to choose healthy, balanced food most of the time.** You can read books on nutrition until the cows come home, but a good place to begin is here, starting with Chapter 3, "Balanced Diet 101—Teen Style."

3. **Get close to nature!** (At least in what you eat.) The less processed the food, the healthier. That means fresh vegetables, fruits, whole-grain breads, lean meats and chicken, and low-fat dairy products.

4. **Enjoy your food.** Food is one of life's great pleasures, and eating is fun! Don't make yourself miserable about it—that's the first step toward restrictive eating and an obsessive relationship with food.

5. **Eat when you're hungry; stop eating when you're full.** Watch out—this is the toughest step of all. Humans are born knowing when they're hungry—by the time we're teens, most of us have stopped paying attention to our body's clues.

"That's it?" you ask. "All I have to do is pay attention to what I eat, understand what makes me healthy, choose less-processed foods, enjoy eating, and eat when—and only when—I'm hungry?"

Basically, yes. Of course there are other little bits (like the importance of breakfast, vitamins, healthy "good fats," and so on) but that's the main plan. If you stick to these five things, I promise you'll eat better, feel better, and look better.

By the way, throughout it all, remember that this is *your* body! You need the flexibility to eat well sometimes, and sometimes not, and incorporate your own tastes and desires into your own diet.

She Sez

"Know that your body is you, it's the closest relationship you'll ever have. It's your number one priority, and it's important to just listen to it."

—Hannah, age 18

What? No Breakfast?

I know, you never have time for breakfast, you would rather sleep that extra 10 minutes in the morning, you can't choke down anything but a glass of juice, and what's the big deal anyway?

Actually, it is a big deal. When you don't eat breakfast, you're running on empty. You get really hungry even if you can't feel it. Your blood sugar drops. You start to crave sugars. You feel edgy, nervous, torked off, maybe depressed. When you go for the donuts or Coke or other empty sugar and fat globules just pretending to be food, your blood sugar goes up fast, then crashes, and you're left feeling sleepy and dog-tired.

Your body needs both quick-energy and slow, long-release energy foods in the morning. Otherwise, there you are, just about mid-morning, trying not to snooze through your English class. All this can be avoided by just eating breakfast.

PHAT Fact

Breakfasts and lunches that are high in protein help power you through the day. Dinners that are high in carbohydrates and lower in protein help you relax and prep you for sleeping.

Breaking That Fast

The best breakfast has three parts: grain, dairy, and fruit:

✧ What's wrong with cereal and milk? It gets you down the road. Add a piece of fruit for flavor and fiber.

✧ Scramble a quick egg, add toast and a glass of juice.

✧ Try peanut butter (it's not just for lunch) and banana slices on an English muffin with a glass of milk.

✧ Go wild and whip up some fresh blueberry pancakes. (Okay, save that idea for the weekend.)

Bizarre Breakfasts

Here are a few ideas for breakfast when you have no time, the only fruit in the house is a soft, brown banana, the muffins are moldy, and your whole body groans, "Cereal, again?"

✧ Think protein. What's wrong with last night's pizza, chicken, spaghetti, or steak?

✧ How about a high-protein shake? Try $^3/_4$ cup soymilk, yogurt, frozen fruit, ice (and maybe a few tablespoons of protein powder). This shake takes less than five minutes to make, and you can take it "to go" if you're late.

She Sez

"Lunch is my biggest meal of the day. I make sure there's frozen stuff like tofu chicken nuggets and frozen peas and carrots in the freezer. I heat them up before I leave home in the morning and then eat them cold at lunch."

—Hannah, age 18

Lunch on the Run

You don't have time to pack a lunch, you can't stand the goop in the school cafeteria, so you head to the local pizza joint or sit down for a burger and fries. Or, you simply skip lunch.

Here are some ideas instead:

- ✧ Pack a lunch the night before. Go for bean salads, a roll on the side, yogurt; anything to get you out of the PBJ, apple, Snapple rut.

- ✧ If you eat in the cafeteria, go for the soup (as long as it's not made with cream). Soups are the great-undiscovered surprise because most cafeterias make them fresh. They tend to taste good!

- ✧ While we're in the cafeteria, forget the steam table goop. And forget the fry counter. (My friend Milo once said to the short-order cook, "May I have a little extra oil on that fried egg?" He didn't realize she was being sarcastic, and she was so sarcastic that she simply thanked him and gravely ate it—swimming in grease.)

- ✧ While we're *still* in the cafeteria, work the beginning and end of the line—salads at the beginning, fruit at the end.

✧ At the local pizza joint, get a salad with dressing on the side (so they don't drown it in goop) and then *don't* order the extra cheese. Remember that veggies are healthy, and skip the pepperoni, sausage, olives, and extra cheese. Pizza crust is good for you—it's a good source of filling, low-fat, carbohydrates.

✧ If it's available near your school, try going out for Asian food—Thai, Vietnamese, Chinese, and if your budget can stand it, the healthiest of all, Japanese.

Snack Attack!

Why do you want a snack? Well, because you're hungry! Your body needs food more often because you're growing so fast—you need those calories and nutrients to keep you going.

PHAT Fact

Wow! Great news! Chocolate is actually good for you! Chocolate is a good source of iron, zinc, calcium, and potassium. And, cocoa butter—chocolate's fat—is metabolized like a "good," heart-healthy fat (rather than a "bad" sat fat).

What makes a good snack? I know: a Big Mac and fries! Nachos! A slice of pie and a Coke! ... Wait! No! Stop! *Wrong!* Just because it's a snack doesn't mean it should be fast, greasy, fatty, sugary food. Most snack foods fill you up but don't have the right nutrients to keep you going.

Here's my general rule about snacking: A snack doesn't have to be "snack food." Food is food, and if you're relying on snacks to get you through the day, snacking on healthful foods will help power you up.

PHAT Fact

Graze! Snack between meals! Your body likes a steady supply of food—it absorbs nutrients better than when it gets it in solid lumps. "Grazers" are also less likely to overeat.

Getting a Knack for Healthy Snacks

If you remember number three of the Basic Eating Plan (eat close to nature), you're most of the way there to healthy snacking. Here are some items to sneak onto the family shopping list:

✧ String cheese. A lot of little kids adore string cheese. It's still fun! And it's got that calcium thing goin' on.

✧ An avocado sliced in half with a lemon squeezed over it and pepper, eaten with a spoon.

✧ Angel food cake (with strawberries or blueberries or raspberries or any berries or sliced nectarines ...) topped with low-fat whipped cream or nothing at all ... yum yum yum ....

✧ Popcorn—microwaved or airpopped—skip the butter. Groovy California kids sometimes sprinkle popcorn with herbs and spices (like oregano or paprika) and even brewer's yeast for a savory, healthy treat.

✧ Baked potato chips. Skip the no-fat chips—they're not good for you.

✧ Peanut butter on a rice cracker.

- ✧ A soy or veggie hot dog—a great hit of protein.
- ✧ Tortilla chips with salsa. Fresh salsa is best—all those fresh tomatoes!
- ✧ Shakes made with ice milk or frozen yogurt and skim milk or soy milk, fruit juice, sliced bananas, or strawberries.

What About Dinner?

Food is best enjoyed when you're sharing it with other people, so it's pretty sad that most families don't eat together anymore. If your family does, congratulations! If you don't, think about suggesting that your family eat together at least a couple meals a week.

PHAT Fact

The closer to dinner, the fewer calories your snack should contain. Or Mom will be right—you will fill up. An hour before dinner, try a piece of fruit. Ten minutes before dinner, better grab the carrot sticks.

Foods for Alertness, Foods for Sleep

If you've eaten well throughout the day, you won't be so starving at dinnertime that you need to scarf it all down and then lie on the floor groaning with your jeans unbuttoned. It's actually harder to sleep on a very full stomach than it is when you've eaten moderately.

The amount you eat is not the only thing that affects your sleep. Certain foods do, too. Some foods are high in carbohydrates that contain an amino acid called tryptophan that help make you sleepy. When you've got to rest up for that big test or game tomorrow, try these snooze foods: pasta, dairy, soy products, seafood, meats, poultry, and whole grains.

Other foods and beverages, those containing caffeine, wake you up or keep you up. They speed up your nervous system and raise your adrenaline, which increases your heart rate and your breathing rate and powers up your digestive system. They set you on a jagged course—high energy now, crash a little later. Caffeine usually affects your body for about six hours. Experts recommend that teens should keep their caffeine consumption to 100 milligrams a day, or roughly the amount in a cup of coffee.

What else has caffeine? Instant coffee has about half the caffeine of a cup of regular coffee. A 12-ounce can of Mountain Dew has 55 milligrams of caffeine, various flavors and brands of cola range from 35 to 45 milligrams, and a cup of tea has 35 milligrams. Then there's the truly important question: Does chocolate have caffeine in it? Well, yes, but not very much. Two chocolate-chip cookies only have about 5 milligrams of caffeine, and a chocolate bar has about 10 milligrams. So don't worry, that hot chocolate in the evening will actually help you snooze, not lose sleep.

PHAT Fact

Turn off the TV while you eat! When it's on, you can't fully pay attention to what you eat, enjoy your food, or notice when you're hungry and full (the Basic Eating Plan). Important show? Tape it for later.

PHAT Fact

Love tea, hate the jitters? Drink herb tea or, if you love the zippy stuff, only drink tea made from the tea bag's second use—most of the caffeine is used in the first cup.

"Want French Fries with That?" Health*ier* Fast Food

Then there's that favorite place: the fast-food joint. At McDonald's, Wendy's, Taco Bell, and Burger King, nutrient-depleted, high-fat foods (and foods high in the worst kinds of fats—saturated fats and hydrogenated fats and oils) tend to be the usual menu items. Here are a few general tips to avoid the unhealthy fast-food trap:

◇ You're in luck! At least you'll know what you're eating. Because so many people are concerned about health, weight, calories, fat, and related issues, most fast-food restaurants offer healthier options and, if you ask for it, a little booklet that lists the nutrients in each of their products.

◇ Don't supersize it. A regular serving size at a fast-food place is often pretty close to a Food Guide Pyramid serving size, but if you go for the jumbo, you're supersizing the fats, too.

◇ Think twice about ordering that second burger or hot dog. A Big Mac is 46 percent fat, a Wendy's chocolate-chip cookie is 37 percent fat, a Carl's Junior breakfast burrito is 54 percent fat—not to mention the mega-calories.

✧ Look for key words like "broiled" and "heart healthy." It's not like eating sawdust and stale water—they taste yummy, too!

Feastin' at the Food Court

When you're at the mall and starving from all the energy you've spent on bargain-hunting, the usual choice for food is the international food court. At first glance, everything here seems unhealthy and about as far away from nature as you can get. Not true!

✧ Hit the baked potato stand (but watch what you put on it).

✧ If you're eating Mexican, go heavy on the salsa, light on the chips.

✧ Munching Italian? Pasta is very healthy—just go light on the heavy cream sauces (choose marinara sauce instead).

✧ You really don't want to know what they put in those hot dogs.

✧ There's often a stand where you can get grilled chicken and salads. Mmmmmm ... makes me hungry just thinking about it.

PHAT Fact

Eat slowly. Your stomach is kinda dumb. It needs to be full for about 20 minutes before it informs your brain. Give it time. Chew, chew, chew, and swallow. Sip water. Repeat.

59

The Least You Need to Know

✧ Pay attention, understand healthy food, eat close to nature, enjoy eating, and eat when—and only when—you're hungry.

✧ Eat both quick-release and slow-release energy foods in the morning.

✧ You need healthy snacks to keep energized throughout the day.

✧ The best dinners are at the table, *not* in front of the TV.

✧ Certain foods make you sleepy. Use them wisely!

✧ Even fast-food restaurants usually have healthier options.

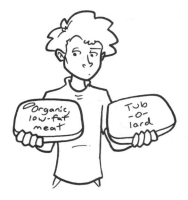

Chapter 5

Changes and Choices in Food

In This Chapter

✧ Making big and little changes

✧ Working with your family to eat better

✧ Tips for doing the family shop

✧ Cooking up a storm!

✧ Organic food and vegetarianism—your choice

This chapter is about changes and choices. Sometimes I read a book or listen to somebody talk and I get so inspired that I swear I'm going to change my ways, become a different person, and live a wonderful, healthful, good life for ever and ever. I'll eat protein in the morning, quit coffee, wash my face the right way every day, and always tell the truth (because every time I don't I mess everything up so bad!).

Then, it happens: I slip up. I don't follow through, or I only follow through halfway. I've learned that making big changes is really, really, really hard; it usually happens through a series of little choices. That's what this chapter is about—small choices you can take to make long term changes in your eating.

When Your Family Makes Lousy Food Choices

People have the best chance to make consistently healthful food choices when they live with families who support their choices and are involved in eating healthfully themselves. So what do you do when your whole family has food issues, eats fried and frozen foods constantly, stocks the house with processed cheese and heavily sugared cereal, and thinks that the color green looks good on trees and redheads, but not on the plate?

You could: A) Change families, B) Try to change your family, or C) Ask for support while you try to change yourself. Option A is probably not feasible. (Plus Mom plays the best music, and Dad rarely complains when you get the bathmat sopping during your shower. That, and you love each other.) But Options B and/or C are possible—in most cases. It all depends on your family and how you present it.

You're not with your family all the time, and you have lots of opportunities to make your own food choices. A lot of times, kids and teens feel that food choices are the *only* choices they get to make! You can always do it on your own. Nevertheless, having support from your family, and living in a family where good, healthy food is available, makes eating healthy much easier. When you're trying to change your family's choices of food, remember these tips:

✧ Focus on your own changes first—and start out of the house if you need to.

✧ Sit down with your parents and tell them that you're interested in eating more healthfully. Be specific about the kind of support you're asking for, for instance: "I'd like to keep more whole-grain cereal and dark green vegetables in the house" or "I want to put some tofu in my lunch."

✧ If you already feed meals to your little sisters or brothers, make your "healthful" changes slowly and silently.

You can help their health without them knowing about it!

✧ Take responsibility for some of the shopping or cooking and then actually do it. "I'll make the salad tonight, okay?"

✧ Nobody likes a loudmouthed convert. Once you've made changes to your diet, don't get all obnoxious about it. It's better to lead by example instead.

When You're the Family Shopper

If you do some of your family's food shopping, you're not alone. A lot of teens do. If you're interested in improving what you eat, shopping for the family is a great opportunity. It's much easier to change your (and your family's) eating habits when you're the one piling that shopping cart high and lugging home the loot.

Shopping can be a blast or a drag. In this section, I'll give you some hints to make the supermarket less a mystery and an easier experience.

He Sez

"When I got my license, I started doing the big family shop once a week. I started buying all organic food. My parents didn't feel strongly about eating organic and they were concerned about the money, but after a while they decided they like eating healthy."

—Jake, age 17

It's the Food, the Whole Food, and Nothing but the Food

If you have trouble choosing food or you generally get too much because it all looks so good, try eating before shopping. If you're hungry, you'll either have a hard time controlling your buying or you'll crave—and restrict yourself—so hard that you'll pass the important stuff by and wander out of the store with a single low-fat yogurt and a diet soda.

Making a List and Checking It Twice

If, like me, you sometimes get baffled and confused in large spaces like supermarkets, it's best to go armed with a list. True "list specialists" say that the best way to organize your list is to put all the dairy together, all the vegetables together, all the meat together, and so on, so you're not running around the store. This is a great idea—for people who like that kind of organization. Even if the idea of planning your trip up and down the aisles gives you the heebie jeebies, it does help to have a list of some kind.

Looking at Labels

When you're shopping in a supermarket, check out the labels that are on every box, bottle, and can. They show the size of a serving (which usually is a lot smaller than you think) plus every major nutrient, vitamin, and mineral in the food.

Glancing at the fat, sugar, and calorie content can be helpful (if you want a food that's not mostly made of fat, for instance, look for a big difference between the number of total calories and the number of fat calories). The ingredient list can also be useful. But what's even more helpful than the label, sometimes, is the little box that sums up all the nutrients.

What's the Definition?

About a decade ago, food regulators came up with a set of standard definitions to make sure that food manufacturers are consistent when it comes to letting consumers know what they're buying and eating. Don't ever be too impressed. I just saw a package of raisins that had "Fat-Free" on the bag. Raisins have *never* had any fat!

Here are a few clues to some of the definitions:

✧ **Low-fat.** It contains 3 grams of fat or less per serving.

✧ **Low saturated fat.** It contains 1 gram or less of saturated fat ("bad" fat) per serving.

✧ **Low-calorie.** It contains 40 calories or less per serving.

✧ **Reduced.** This is a nutritionally altered product, and it contains at least 25 percent less of whatever they say is "reduced."

✧ **Fat (or anything else)-free.** The product contains virtually no fat (or anything else mentioned).

✧ **Light.** This can mean one of two things: Either it has one third the calories or half the fat of the "nonlight" version, or it can refer to the sodium content.

PHAT Fact

If you're into reading labels, that's cool. If you really aren't into it, don't worry, you can still eat well. Basic rule: The less it's been messed with, the better for you it is.

Trimming the Fat Without Bulging the Budget

Guess what? Eating well can actually save you money. This may seem hard to believe! If you go to the store and look at the outrageous prices on organic vegetables, for instance, you might go screaming to the frozen dinner aisle or out of the store and down the block to grab another burger and fries. But done right, you can save your money (and your family's money) for that CD you've been craving or that cool new hat. Think about this:

✧ If you're in charge of buying your own lunches and snacks, you can save a boodle by packing your own (even "expensive" items like gourmet fruit leather or roll-ups and prepared salads!).

✧ Eating closer to the earth helps save you money. Buying meat, vegetables, and fruit to prepare yourself—even fancy meat, vegetables, and fruit—is a lot cheaper in the long run than buying packaged, processed products. This makes sense when you consider that you're not paying for all that cooking, processing, and packaging.

✧ Buy in bulk. Buying fresh food in bulk (fruit and vegetables) doesn't always work unless you're throwing a party or feeding a large group of monkeys (sometimes this feels like the same thing). But when it comes to grains and beans and potatoes and things, the bigger the package, the cheaper the food usually works out to be.

Becoming a Kitchen God or Goddess

If you want to make changes in your eating, particularly if your family is lagging a little behind, it helps to be able to cook. Although cooking is a skill, it's also an enormous amount of fun. Remember being a kid and playing in mud, making sandcastles, and creating Play-Doh animals? Cooking can be a wonderful way for teens and adults to play, long after you've left childhood behind. For many people, cooking is an enjoyable creative outlet. Cooking for your family is a great way to take on more responsibilities; plus, everything tastes better when you've made it yourself.

He Sez

"Cooking means you get to taste a lot of good food. It's satisfying to feel more independent. I like being able to fool around with different things, and food is a good way to do it. Like in art, you get to be creative with it, but you also get to eat it."

—Josh, age 14

Whether you're just beginning to cook or you've been cooking for a long time, there's always room to hone your skills. Ready for some tips?

⬧ Take it slow. As you build up your cooking chops, don't expect to be able to do everything at once. Concentrate on learning to make a few wonderful dishes.

⬧ Select recipes that use very few ingredients, don't take a lot of time to prepare, and don't involve a lot of chopping, straining, sifting, or other preparation.

⬧ Give yourself enough time. Watch cooking shows for inspiration and to work up an appetite, but don't expect to be able to do it like the experts. Plan on tripling the preparation time on everything you see.

⬧ Plan ahead. Decide what you want to prepare, check ingredients, go to the store, and *then* begin to make your delicacy.

⬧ Use recipes as a way to inspire yourself, not as a complete set of rules. The more creative you get, the more fun you'll have! True chefs talk about "listening" to the ingredients. Don't be afraid to play! Experiment with new foods, new ingredients, and new ways to prepare them.

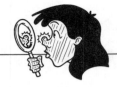

Beautiful? NOT!

Although it's a great idea to get creative with the recipe when you're cooking a meal, it's best to stick to the recipe when you're baking—baking is like a chemistry experiment, and we all know what can happen with a chemistry experiment gone wrong (think Frankenstein!).

✧ Taste the food as you go. How do you know how much salt, how much oregano, or how much vinegar you need if you don't taste it? Just don't eat it all before it's ready!

✧ Fail. Burn things, over-salt things, have things stick to the pan. The only way you'll really learn to cook is to get in there and do it.

Organics—They're Not Just for Hippies Anymore

Organic food tastes better. It's better for you, and it's better for the enviroment. It used to be that organics were only available in specialty health-food stores and cooperative (co-op) grocery markets. But not anymore. You may have noticed separate sections in your grocery store for organic food—especially organic produce and grains. Organic foods are grown with only natural, nonsynthetic substances and are better for your body. They are grown only in safe, healthy soil, using natural fertilizers, without synthetic pesticides. They also might be higher in nutrients, and—bonus points—they taste great!

She Sez

"I only eat organic. This is mainly based on loving my body and not wanting to contaminate it. If I eat junk food, I don't feel good physically. I focus on eating pure and healthy and good."

—Hannah, age 18

Moving Toward Vegetarianism

Some statistics say as many as 25 percent of all teens are vegetarians or seriously interested in becoming one. Vegetarianism (not eating meat products) can be a healthy option, so long as you understand how to keep your diet balanced and aren't using it as an excuse to begin restricted eating.

Why Teens Become Vegetarians

There are almost as many reasons that teens become vegetarians as there are places they pierce their bodies (and that's a lot!). Some of the major reasons include:

- ✧ **Concern for animals.** It's no secret that animals are often kept in cruel conditions.

- ✧ **Health.** Vegetarians eat far less "bad" sat fats than non-vegetarians, and they have a lower risk for heart disease and some types of cancer.

- ✧ **Environmental issues.** Producing meat takes a huge amount of resources (land, water, and grain) and produces a lot of pollution. Some say it takes up to three times the amount of energy resources to feed a meat-eater than it does to feed a vegetarian.

Your reasons may include any or all of these, and your vegetarianism may also change over time.

Vegetarianism—It's a Tricky Thing

Be careful of eliminating foods from your diet without adding other ones back in. "The more teens restrict their diets,
the more dangerous. Becoming a vegetarian could be a warning signal for restrictive eating," says Stanford University nutritionist Jo Ann Hattner. She says, "The more vegan you are,
the more education you need." Hattner also warns that some
teens have difficulty tolerating foods—such as meat—once
they've taken them out of their diet.

The Least You Need to Know

❖ Making long-term changes is hard; take baby steps.

❖ Lead by example. Work to change your own eating;
then work with your family.

❖ Cook! It's fun, it's creative, it's challenging, and it's
healthy.

❖ Eating organic food is excellent for your health (and
tasty, too).

❖ Vegetarianism is a good option—so long as you do it
carefully.

Part 3

Safe and Effective Weight Loss

Okay, okay, you're not thrilled with those extra pounds on your tum or your bum. If you're like many, many teens, you're concerned about losing weight. But it's tricky! Losing weight the wrong way can make you ill, damage your body, and ... here's the kicker ... actually make you gain weight!

This section will help you get control of your weight and your eating—safely. There's info on weight loss and weight maintenance, and what to do when you're struggling with eating issues. Dive on in!

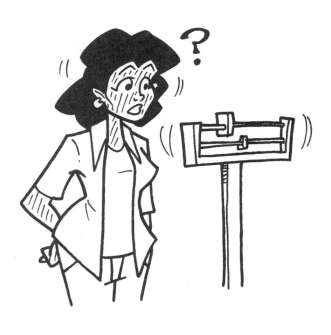

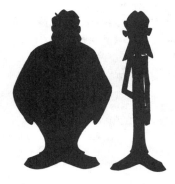

Chapter 6

Fat and Thin— Trimming the Shape You're In

In This Chapter

✧ Understanding why people get fat

✧ Assessing your own weight and shape

✧ The basic diet modification plan for teens

✧ When you need to gain weight

Why can some people swallow the refrigerator without gaining an ounce, and others merely look at a piece of pie and feel their waistlines growing? In this chapter, we'll look at a very heavy issue—weight! Whether you're average size, overweight, obese, skinny, or anything in between, you're probably concerned about your weight (just about everybody in our society is). To become the right weight for your body, you need to know a bit about how it all works.

Whatcha Mean, Fat?

Forget about the word "fat." There's no clear definition of it. And even more, forget about the word "thin." It's bogus. Too often "thin" really means "skinny." And skinny is not always healthy.

The word "overweight," in the medical sense, means you weigh more than the standard weight and height charts recommend. But if you're a big-boned person who works out a lot and are truly buff, you might weigh a lot more than the charts recommend. Yet if you're tiny-boned, out of shape, and flabby, you could still fit into the recommended slot on the standard charts.

Remember that the important thing isn't the word "fat" or "thin" or anything else—aim to be *trim*. Trim = fit, with the right weight for your height and bone structure.

Media Images

Trim is healthy. Skinny—having an ultra-low amount of body fat because you're undernourished—is not. What's hot in bodies changes and, unfortunately, right now, for girls and women, toothpick-skinny is in, despite the fact that there aren't too many natural toothpicks out there.

Body styles change frequently—sometimes thin is in; at other times in history, buff, buxom, or bigger is better. It's hard to fight against current styles, but you'll be happier (and healthier!) if you try to have the best body in the world—for you. Your body has a best inside it. What's best for you is based on your body type, your temperament, and your metabolism.

Fat and Thin and in Between

Your metabolism and temperament have a great deal to do with your weight.

Your Metabolism

Your metabolism is the rate at which your body burns calories and turns them into energy. Some people have a naturally fast metabolism, while other people's metabolisms are slower. When you exercise regularly, your metabolism speeds up and you naturally burn more calories. When you're depressed or just hanging out in front of the TV every evening, your metabolism slows. The slower the metabolism, the less energy burned, and the more fat you'll tend to retain on those bones of yours.

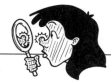

Beautiful? NOT!

Danger: Are you starting to restrict your diet? Restriction leads to misery, eating disorders, and/or weight gain!

Your Energy!

Some people are naturally easygoing and slow-moving. You know the type (you might even be one!): From the time they're babies, not much throws them, and they pass through life at a relaxed pace. Other people (like me!) have a ton of energy, much of it nervous. They fidget, they worry, and they bounce around. A person with high energy will naturally burn more calories just going about the daily business of eating, breathing, working, and sleeping. You can't change your basic temperament or energy—it's part of who you are. You can work with it, however.

It's Mom and Dad's Fault

Just like your hair, your eyes, and your skin color (and tendency to break out, as you'll see in Chapter 14, "The Skin You're In"), your weight is tied to the weight of your parents and grandparents. And it's not just about what the family eats (although that certainly has a huge impact). Some people, and some families, are bigger than other families, but no matter what your genes say, you can be healthier, more toned, more energetic—and by getting *there,* you'll likely be trimmer as well.

Why Do People Get Overweight?

People get overweight for a lot of reasons. Some of it is genetic—your inborn body type, your basic metabolism, and your temperament all have a huge influence right from the start. But all people can be trim and fit—why aren't they? Here are the basic reasons:

✧ **They eat more calories than they use up.** In other words, they simply eat too much food for their bodies.

✧ **They eat unhealthful food.** If you eat a lot of "empty food," that is, high-fat, high-sugar foods without a lot of other vitamins, minerals, proteins, complex carbohydrates, or other good things to recommend them, you'll tend to get overweight. You can't just count calories! A calorie does *not* equal a calorie no matter how you slice it.

✧ **They don't move that lovely body.** Exercise not only burns up calories, it also is the only thing that can reset your metabolism to burn at a higher level.

PHAT Fact

Fat forever? Scientists once believed that heavy teens were doomed to be fat forever. Not so! It's hard to change, but many heavy people become—and stay—trim and fit for the rest of their lives.

Why Do People Get Obese?

Obese is a medical term that means you weigh more than 120 percent of the recommended weight on the chart for your height. People get obese for all the reasons people get overweight, plus more. For a very few people, the little thing in the brain that tells them they're full doesn't work at all.

For another set of very few people, the body doesn't metabolize food effectively. These people need medical care to help correct their obesity. But for more than 90 percent of the population, nothing like that is going on.

Genetics plays a huge role in obesity, too. If one of your parents is obese, you have a 40 percent chance of becoming obese, too. If both are, your chances go higher.

PHAT Fact

"Nutrient-dense" food contains a lot of nutrition for the smallest amount of calories. You need a lot of nutrients. So go for the density!

Do You Need to Lose Weight?

Don't be ruled by the scale or the chart! Determine whether you need to adjust your eating (and exercise) habits for weight control by looking at, and listening to, your body's warning signals.

- ✧ Are you tired all the time? How is your energy? When you walk up a flight of stairs, are you panting and huffing and puffing when you arrive?

- ✧ Has your doctor suggested that you need to be more fit?

- ✧ Do you have diabetes, high blood pressure, bad back, or aching knees? Is your weight impacting your health?

- ✧ How's your muscle tone? Are you flabby? Can you "pinch an inch"?

Here are some reasons *not* to lose weight:

✧ You wear a size eight but you really like the number six better than the number eight.

✧ All your friends are thinner than you. (They might have smaller bones or a different body type.)

✧ You just know that if you were 10 pounds thinner, your life would be different. (I promise you up, down, and sideways that it wouldn't make a big difference.)

Doin' Something About It

Now for the bad news ....

All the nutrition experts and pediatricians strongly recommend against weight reduction diets for teens. That's right—no diets!

Okay, wait, don't slam the book shut and throw it to the ground! I'm not going to strand you out there! Everybody I talked to gave me a lecture on the dangers of dieting for teens—dieting compromises your health, makes you feel weak and irrational, and might actually affect how tall you'll grow.

But teens do diet and will diet, so the best I can do is tell you how to diet safely and diet effectively. But I warn you, don't plan to lose 10 pounds by your hot date next week. First of all, it won't work without making you very sick, and second, you would be "fat" again just in time for the second hot date.

Get This: Diets Are Fattening!

Most people who lose weight gain it all back again—unless they change how they eat and their relationship with food. I promise you this: If you change your focus from weight to fitness and health, you will firm up, look terrific, and feel great!

Here's the medical rationale: Your body uses fat as a back-up reserve. It's the same way a camel drinks a lot of water when it hits an oasis so that it can walk for miles and days in the desert without getting dehydrated. It lives off its reserves.

Any time you prevent your body from getting the nutrients it is used to (like when you go on a restrictive or crash diet), it basically goes into starvation mode, and begins to do what it's designed to do—it lives off your reserve fat. That's what makes you thinner. Then, the starvation mode makes you want to replace all those fat stores, and your appetite increases. Your body says, "Ooh baby, I better store up more fat just in case this happens again!" and all of a sudden you can't stop eating until you're heavier than when you started.

PHAT Fact

Results of a recent four-year study of 692 teenage girls show that those who dieted during high school years actually gained more weight than those who didn't!

Here are a couple of points:

- ✧ Most diets don't work the way you want them to (it might be easy to lose weight temporarily, but it's hard to lose weight forever).
- ✧ No matter how much you weigh and how much you want to lose, the only true solution is the same. And that's what the rest of this chapter—and the whole of the next chapter—is about!

Losing It!

There's no real secret to losing weight and keeping it off. Here are the basic principals of getting trim:

1. Eat nutritious, nutrient-dense food in smaller portions.

2. Exercise.

3. Eat healthy snacks.

PHAT Fact

It's normal for both girls and guys to get a little pudgy during adolescence. Blame it on hormones. Blame it *all* on hormones!

Gimme a Recipe!

Of course you want a recipe. Everybody does—that's why all those diet books sell millions. There's no recipe here, but I do have a series of suggestions.

But first get out your "Looking Great" Journal and your calendar. Write down today's date. Now write down what date it will be a month from now.

The First Week

The first week is your week to gather information. This week, you're just learning more about your own relationship with food.

Read Chapters 3, "Balanced Diet 101—Teen Style," 4, "Eating on the Run—Eating for Your Lifestyle," and 5, "Changes and Choices in Food," to begin understanding more about nutrition and food choices. As you read, begin to watch what you eat—I mean watch it; don't do anything about it yet. Make some entries in your "Looking Good" Journal.

Here are some suggestions for topics:

✧ What makes you overeat?

✧ What do you love about food, and what foods do you love?

✧ What do you like about being overweight?

✧ If you've dieted before, write about what the experience was like. Did you enjoy it? Did it work? What was hard? What went wrong? What was scary? What was successful?

You won't come to any conclusions, but you might get a better idea of where you are with food and dieting.

Going for It: Weeks Two, Three, and Four

Now you'll start to take action. The following list of suggestions is huge—do the best you can; small changes add up.

Watching Calories

If you can manage to reduce your intake of calories by only 250 a day, you're guaranteed to lose weight. Wait! I don't mean count every calorie or even keep a food journal! Just pay attention to the food, educate yourself about which foods have a lot of calories and which don't, and make your choices accordingly.

Eat Fat—Good Fat!

Pay attention to fat, but don't just cut it all out of your diet. Don't get caught in the "no-fat low-fat" trap. Teen brains need fat! Healthy fat! When you eat a lot of "bad" saturated fats and hydrogenated oils and when you cut out "good" polyunsaturated fats, you're asking for trouble.

Love Them Veggies!

If you're cutting out 250 calories a day, you're gonna be hungry. Replace those calories with high-fiber foods—fruits and vegetables. Vegetables are ...

❖ Incredibly nutrient-dense.

❖ "Free foods"—meaning you can eat as much as you want without thinking about it or counting calories.

❖ Cancer-fighting (if you're thinking long term).

❖ Never boring. Vegetables come in lots of varieties; you can always try a different one.

❖ Full of fiber and delightfully complex carbohydrates.

PHAT Fact

Fiber makes you fuller faster.

Skip Dessert

No, not every dessert! But really think about whether you need, want, and ache for that particular dessert at that particular time. Will a beautiful orange, fresh and juicy, do as well? If you do have dessert, don't punish yourself by avoiding "real" food. You still need the nutrients. And indulging yourself now doesn't mean you've fallen off the wagon, that's it, it's over, you've failed. You have choices again every time you eat!

Don't Skip Meals

Eat every meal, and eat frequent healthy snacks. Eating small amounts more often helps you digest your food and keeps you from getting so hungry that you need to pig out.

She Sez

"I believe in being nice to myself. Sometimes instead of eating I actually take myself to the movies or just buy a big bottle of expensive water."

—Christie, age 18

Banish the Scales

Stop weighing yourself every day. Hide the scale in the closet, put a pile of dirty laundry on top of it, pile a bunch of old coats on top of that, and booby trap the door so a pile of books falls on your head if you open the closet door. Your body has a natural weight fluctuation (especially if you're female)—some days you might have more waste in you, you might have more water retention, and so on. If you weigh yourself every day, you won't be able to see the big picture.

Creative Indulgence

Find other ways to indulge yourself. (Use your "Looking Great" Journal to list three ways of pampering your sensual side.)

Focus on Water

Sometimes when you think you're hungry, you're actually thirsty. When you get dehydrated, you feel tired, so you reach for food to boost your energy. Really, you need water. Experts recommend six to eight glasses of water a day. Eight glasses a day is a lot of water—it means you have to have a glass of water almost every time you think about it. Water helps flush the poisons, keeps you feeling satisfied, and makes your skin look great. (There's more on this in Chapter 14.)

PHAT Fact

A glass of OJ has 120 calories. You can lose weight by switching your beverage of choice from soda or juice to water.

Limit Sodas and Caffeine

Nutritionists recommend that teens drink only 200 milligrams of caffeine a day or less. That's one cup of coffee. Why? Well, caffeine is a diuretic (there goes all that water you're drinking); plus it leaches valuable calcium from your bones and makes you jittery. And even noncaffeine sodas have phosphoric acid in them—not great for you at all.

Slow Down and Eat Smaller Portions

Just like your mama said, chew your food thoroughly. Wanna fill your plate? Get your family to use smaller plates!

Make Wise Substitutions

How about extra salsa instead of extra sour cream on that burrito? You know what to do.

Eat a Variety of Foods

Try new things. The human body gets tired of eating the same foods over and over again. If your mind or body feels restricted, it will rebel.

Focus on Nutrition and Exercise

Losing weight will be a side effect. Have patience in losing a half pound to one pound a week; this is the most effective way of all to lose weight, because it's long term! Whether you're trying to lose a couple of pounds or a lot more than that, it's got to be gradual or it just will not work.

Move Your Lovely Body

Exercise. This chapter is not about that—check out the chapters in Part 4, "Work That Body! Safe Fitness for Teens."

Week Five

Get out your "Looking Great" Journal. Weigh yourself. Write the weight down and compare it to where you started. See some progress? I told you so!

Gotta Gain Weight?

No chapter about weight would be complete without tips for gaining weight:

- ✧ Up the calories! You should try for between an additional 200 to 1,000 calories a day.

- ✧ Go for the carbo load. Your additional calories should mostly be pasta, bread, potatoes, and rice—complex carbohydrates.

- ✧ Your snacks should be healthy—and you should eat a lot of them. Try bread, granola, fruit, and so on.

- ✧ Drink more milk and more fruit juices.

- ✧ Weight training can help bulk you up.

The Least You Need to Know

✧ Your weight is based on your eating and exercise habits, your temperament, your body type, your metabolism, and your genes.

✧ Skinny is out; trim is in. Aim for health, and you'll look great!

✧ Dieting is not recommended for teens. But if you're gonna do it, do it safely.

✧ Yes, you *can* gain weight by upping your calories and exercise.

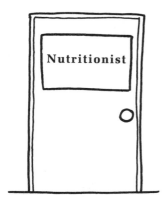

Help and Maintenance

In This Chapter

✧ Losing weight with organizational and community help

✧ Tips for keeping it off

✧ Troubled eating, disordered eating

✧ The truth about smoking, alcohol, drugs, and weight

Food, eating, losing weight—these are all challenging issues. This chapter focuses on the *heavy* stuff.

Even though this is a *thin* chapter, it's filled with *weighty* information, and *larded* with helpful tips. I spent a lot of time *pounding* the keyboard over this one (groan). Okay, don't shoot! I'll stop.

Whys and Why Nots of Weight Loss Organizations

A lot of people make a lot of money off of people who want to lose weight. Just turn on the TV and you'll see ads for diet products and foods, diet organizations, and bogus devices to help you slim down. How do you know who to trust?

Weight-loss organizations, when effective, provide support services and information to people who want or need to lose weight. But watch out—there are a lot of gnarly, not-so-good or ineffective organizations and plans out there. Gimmicks and shortcuts don't work—whether you learn about them through books or through an organized group.

If you feel you're not being successful at losing weight on your own and want to try a weight-loss organization's plan, think about these points before you sign up:

✧ Be leery of any program that sells you their food as a primary part of the program. You might lose weight initially, but you will not keep it off unless—from the beginning—you modify your own food choices. You're gonna be eating real food for the rest of your life, and unless real food is part of your weight loss, you'll regain that weight.

✧ Losing weight should not be expensive. Be careful of any company that charges you a lot of money to lose weight.

✧ There are no quick fixes. Herbs don't do it. Starvation doesn't do it. Papaya juice doesn't do it. Enzymes don't do it. Algae doesn't do it. Protein alone doesn't do it. Carbohydrates alone don't do it. Get the picture? There are no quick fixes. Weight loss is a process!

✧ Effective weight-loss organizations incorporate exercise directly into the eating/dieting plan.

✧ Effective weight-loss organizations include counseling or group meetings into the eating/dieting plan.

✧ Effective weight-loss organizations provide follow-ups. Losing the weight is only the first half of the process. And, realistically, it's the easy half!

PHAT Fact

Food is not your enemy. It is your nourishment.

School, Community, and Friendly Support

You might not have to turn to a for-profit weight loss organization to get the support and help you need to lose weight. Other resources might be available to you. Many schools have support services for losing weight. The best support system is, of course, your parents and friends, *if* they can be supportive of you.

When Friends and Family Fail You

Shh ... I'm gonna tell you a nasty truth. Sometimes the very people you need to be most supportive of you can't be or won't be. Some of them, subconsciously, might even have some sort of interest in keeping you overweight, so they look good in comparison, so you can overeat together, so you don't attain something they feel they can't ... or for other, subconscious reasons.

It can be very disappointing, and can really undermine your confidence and resolve when the people around you are not truly supportive of your changes. People are frightened of change—especially changes (even when they're good changes) in the people around them.

Changing Anyway

Changing your eating patterns is really hard, both physically and emotionally, and it makes a big difference if you have the support of the people around you. If you're not getting what you need, what can you do?

That's one reason why people join organizations like Weight Watchers or go to Overeaters Anonymous groups. The other people in these groups can function as your allies—people who are on your side—at times when your pals, parents, and other relatives, for whatever reason, cannot be.

She Sez

"A lot of girls are worried about what they look like in the cafeteria. The girls say, 'Can you buy this for me so I don't look like I'm buying so much? I don't want to look like a pig.'"

—Arden, age 13

Help from a Nutritionist

You might also contact a nutritionist who can help you make sense of your eating habits.

If you do see a nutritionist, he or she will probably ...

- ✧ Assess what you've been eating.
- ✧ Provide you with suggestions for eating/eating plan.
- ✧ Be somebody who you can check in with about your eating.

Maintaining a Healthy Weight

Losing weight is the easy part (okay, not easy at all, but easier.) No matter what diet you choose (healthy or unhealthy), if you work hard and honestly at it, you'll probably lose weight because you're making an effort, you're focusing on the issue, you're paying attention, you're using your will power.

But you won't keep it off—nobody does—unless you make real changes in your eating habits, you make real changes in your exercise habits, and you continue to pay attention.

So You Got There! Now What?

Okay! Congratulations! You've attained your weight goals! You look mah-valous, dahlink. Whee! Time to celebrate with a gallon of Coke and a dozen donuts! And what about McDonald's? You've been craving those fries and, oh yeah, can you super-size that?

What's happening? Only the dieter's nightmare. Only what will happen if you try to take the pounds off too fast, or in an unhealthy way.

Look, it's normal to want to splurge if you've been feeling deprived. The only real answer is to avoid depriving yourself during the weight loss process. Here are some other tips for keeping the weight off once you're there:

- ✧ Keep making healthy choices in food.

- ✧ Don't forget that, if you blow it, you have a new chance to make a healthy choice in just a few hours, when it's time to eat the next meal.

- ✧ Celebrate your weight loss with rewards other than food: new clothing, a couple of CDs you've been wanting, a long-distance phone call to an old friend. For once and for all, try to separate food from reward.

Backsliding

And what if you do regain some, or all of, the weight? It's hard not to beat yourself up about it. Remind yourself ...

- ✧ The time you spent eating healthy food and exercising is not lost time—you've added to your overall health.

✧ Keep focusing on your health and fitness, and you will gain the strong, fit body you crave.

✧ It takes time to make real change. Be kind to yourself.

✧ If you set yourself up as "bad" when you overeat, you'll punish yourself for being "bad"—and losing control— by eating even more.

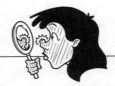

Beautiful? NOT!

Sometimes at the gym you'll see people in the sauna with sweat pants on, trying to lose weight. Not smart. While you do lose water weight through sweating, all you need to do is drink a single glass of water and, voilà!, it's all back.

Eating Troubles and Troubled Eating

Lots of people use food (or the lack of it) to cope with difficult feelings. As my friend Annie says, "Stressed equals desserts spelled backward." If you pig out or binge, or if you restrict your eating because of issues with food or your body, it doesn't necessarily mean you've got an eating disorder— but it might mean that you're miserable about food or hurting yourself with it.

Restrictive Eating and Extreme Eating Issues

There's a kind of large, gray area between "normal" eating and eating disorders such as anorexia and bulimia. Eating disorders are medical conditions, and you have to have certain behaviors and beliefs—including a completely distorted body image—to be diagnosed with one of them. I'll describe them in the following sections.

If you're in this very common gray area, you have issues with eating and food and weight, but your eating is not full-blown "disordered." You might be restricting your eating or practicing "extreme" eating (pigging out). You might be trying fad diets, or just obsessing on your weight, believing that dropping a few pounds will make you happy.

At one time or another in life, most girls and women, and many boys, have restrictive eating or extreme eating and body image issues. Even though they're not technically eating disordered, they're still unhappy and often have unhealthy eating patterns.

Disordered Eating

Sometimes food becomes an addiction and eating—or not eating—becomes the focus of our lives. Eating disorders can happen to people of any age, but teens are particularly at risk—especially bright, accomplished teens. Disordered eating is usually related to control issues, poor body image, and stress.

If you feel that your body or your life is out of control (and think about it, when you're a teen your body *is* surging out of control), it's common to try to control the one area you absolutely can—your eating.

If you feel bad about how your body looks (and face it, with the messages we get from TV, movies, and magazines about what people should look like, most of us have some sort of negative body image), it's common to try to "fix" that bad image by restricting your diet.

If you're under stress (and, realistically, modern life for teens is very stressful), it's common to soothe yourself with food. In the extreme, this soothing can become pigging out or compulsive overeating.

Guys Have Issues, Too

It's not just girls who get anorexic, bulimic, or who overeat compulsively. More and more, people are becoming aware that guys suffer from eating disorders, too. Guys ...

✦ Have a real horror of being fat.

✦ Want to be buff.

✦ Are most likely to express their disorders by taking steroids or supplements and working out obsessively.

Whatcha Mean with All this Nervosa Stuff?

There are three main types of eating disorders:

✦ **Compulsive overeating** (can lead to obesity). Do you pig out? Do you start eating (maybe because you've been restricting your food, or dieting) and can't stop until you're sick? Compulsive overeating comes in all varieties. Mainly, it's compulsive overeating if it's *compulsive* (you can't seem to stop yourself) and it's *overeating* (you're eating more food—a lot more food—than your body needs).

✦ **Anorexia Nervosa** (self-starvation). This is kind of like compulsive under-eating, but being convinced, at the same time, that you're fat, even though you're a walking skeleton. True anorexia is not just about starving yourself. *Anorexia* is an eating disorder characterized by self-starvation because of a distortion of body image.

✦ **Bulimia Nervosa** (binge eating and purging) Bulimia is characterized by cycles of bingeing (overeating) and self-induced purging (vomiting or overuse of laxatives). Bulimics often maintain a normal weight. It's an easy disorder to hide; it's a dangerous disorder to avoid dealing with. Bingeing and purging can have long-term effects on your body, from your teeth to your (ugh) bowel.

✦ **Other eating disorders.** Just because you don't fit neatly into one of the categories above doesn't mean you might not be ill. What if you compulsively overeat and then starve yourself for a few days? Technically, it's not Bulimia, it's not Anorexia, and it may not fit the classic patterns of compulsive overeating. The difficulty is figuring out if you need help with your behavior. Say it's your best friend's birthday party and you eat a lot of cake and the next few days take it easy on the dessert. Is that sick? No! That's normal regulation. But if it's a pattern for you to pig out until you feel sick and then get freaked 'cause you're getting fat so you make yourself throw up, then something *is* going on with your eating.

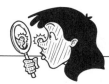

Beautiful? NOT!

Starving yourself robs your body of the nutrients you need to stay healthy: vitamins, mineral, carbohydrates, proteins, and fats. And yes, you do need fat in your diet!

Are You at Risk?

Whether you're a male or a female, you're at risk for developing an eating disorder when you ...

- ✧ Dwell on how you don't meet an unrealistic beauty standard.
- ✧ Put yourself on restrictive diets.
- ✧ Check the scale every day.
- ✧ Work out obsessively.
- ✧ Constantly count calories in your head.
- ✧ Keep strict food journals.
- ✧ Binge compulsively.
- ✧ Use diet drugs to stay thin.
- ✧ Purge through the use of diuretics, laxatives, or vomiting.

PHAT Fact

The American Anorexia/Bulimia Association says 90 percent of all teenagers with eating disorders are female. In the United States, 1 percent of teenage girls suffer from Anorexia.

Professional Counseling—the Big Guns

If you have an eating disorder—or even if you're struggling with restrictive eating—consider getting some help with it. It's almost impossible to "do" eating disorders alone. You can go a variety of ways with this:

❖ Your school might have an educational program about eating disorders (many do).

❖ Read about it on the Net or in the library. You'll feel less panicked the more you know.

❖ A therapist who specializes in body image/eating disorders can help you figure out what's going on underneath and help you get it under control.

Negative Input—Smoking, Drinking, Drugs

There are lots of health reasons to not smoke, drink, or do other drugs, but in this chapter I'm going to stay focused on how using these substances affects your weight. Various drugs have different effects on your weight. Here are some facts:

❖ Smoking cigarettes does not make you lose weight. If you quit smoking, yes, you might gain some weight—

a small amount, and temporarily. So, you can keep smoking and keep off a temporary pound or two and have yellow, wrinkly skin and deep bags under your eyes, have a chronic bad taste in your mouth, smell awful, wake up cranky, damage your lungs, risk cancer, mess up your circulatory system, lose your wind, walk around with stained teeth and stained fingers, and be a slave to the cigarette companies, or ... you can quit smoking or, better yet, don't start.

✧ Marijuana can give you the munchies.

✧ Alcohol has a lot of empty calories. Severe alcoholics are often very thin because they neglect food in favor of alcohol and don't get the nutrients they need. For the casual or social user, alcohol can make you gain weight (think about all those guys with beer bellies).

✧ Speed (amphetamines) used to be prescribed as a weight-loss drug—until they discovered that people might have gotten thinner on them, but they were strung out on the speed, their nerves were shot, and their brain cells were dying. You can lose weight by cutting off your head, too.

✧ Heroin and crack users tend to be thin, too, but it's not a good-looking kind of thin. Stringy, gaunt, unhealthy— no, it's not a good look (to say the least!).

The Least You Need to Know

✧ Beware of weight-loss organizations that don't include exercise and counseling, don't provide follow-up services, and/or cost a lot of money.

✧ Friends and family aren't always supportive.

✧ There's a huge gray region between normal, carefree eating and the obsessive, unhealthy regulation of your diet that characterizes an eating disorder.

✧ Restrictive eating and eating disorders need professional attention.

✧ Smoking, alcohol, and other drugs are not effective—and are very dangerous—ways to lose weight.

Part 4

Work That Body! Safe Fitness for Teens

Exercise—moving that bod of yours—is probably the most important part of improving your looks (and how you feel). These chapters give you the ins and outs, the ups and downs, the long and the short of many types of working out—from the gym to the pool to the track to the floor in front of the TV. You'll get a quick peek into the world of martial arts and dance, too. Oh yeah ... here's where you learn things about taking your heart rate, what to do about a sprain, and how to choose the perfect athletic shoe. It's in the details! So slip into your sweats, and let's take a run at it.

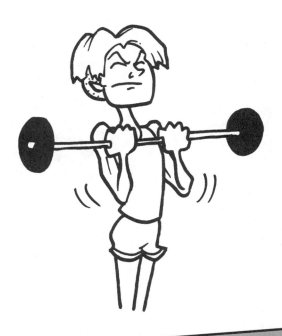

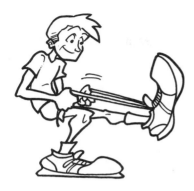

Chapter 8

Setting Up and Exercisin' It!

In This Chapter

✧ The goods on exercise

✧ Things to know before you begin working out

✧ "What do you mean, 'aerobic'?"

✧ Fitting in fitness

✧ Whatcha gonna wear?

What makes you beautiful? Beauty is far more than having even, pretty features or ruggedly handsome looks; true beauty comes from the inside, and there's absolutely nothing more ravishingly gorgeous than a fit person glowing with good health. I'm not talking necessarily buff (but there's nothing wrong with that, either!), just active. This chapter begins focusing your energies on looking great from the inside out through exercise.

So, Why Exercise?

You're overworked at school and overstressed at home; plus, since you've been reading this book, you're spending time focusing on eating well. (Right? Just checking.) Hey, life's crammed enough; the last thing you might want is to add one more thing—such as exercising—to your schedule. So to convince you to try, I've thrown together a list of some of the great things exercising can do for you:

✧ Exercise gives you energy! The time you spend exercising will be paid back in increased energy and a better ability to focus.

✧ Exercise increases your confidence.

✧ Exercise keeps your body fit, gorgeous, and healthy.

✧ It's fun! It feels good! (Okay, okay, it doesn't always feel good at the exact instant, but it sure feels nice later.)

✧ Over the long term, exercise protects your body from brittle bones (osteoporosis), colon cancer, hypertension, and heart disease.

✧ Exercise helps ward off depression and can help lighten existing depression.

✧ (Guys, you can skip this one.) Exercise reduces menstrual cramps and PMS (more on this in Chapter 17, "Attack of the Hormones!").

✧ Exercise, combined with a healthy diet, is an important part of losing weight.

✧ Exercise is an awesome way to love your body.

PHAT Fact

Does exercising really make you hungrier? Not really. Researchers now think the link between working out and wanting to chow down is mostly in your head.

Before You Start ...

Most teens already do some exercise in school, after school, or on their own. But the older teens get, the less likely they are to work out or participate in sports. If you already exercise, keep it up! If you aren't exercising now, begin slowly. The first task is to understand how fit your body is.

Here are some of the questions you should consider:

✧ Are you overweight or obese?

✧ Do you have any ongoing medical problems?

✧ Do you smoke?

✧ When you walk fewer than four miles, are you exhausted?

If you answered "yes" to any of these, check with your doctor. She'll probably recommend beginning with a mild form of exercise (walking or swimming) instead of with a high-level one (running the triathlon or signing up for Capoeira classes—you'll have to read Chapter 12, "Martial Arts—Far Eastern–Style Fitness," if you want to find out what these are!).

More important than what the doctor says, though, is what you feel. As you begin your exercise program, listen carefully to what your body is telling you. And remember that exercise—especially at first—can feel hard (it is!). But pain, dizziness, or nausea are always reasons to s-l-o-w way down or stop.

What Do You Mean, Exercise?

Okay, now that we've gotten the disclaimers out of the way, let's start talking about exercise. There are many ways you can get exercise—the following chapters cover a lot of them—but exercise falls into three main categories: aerobic, strength- and muscle-building, and stretching. Of course, many activities combine two of these types, and many combine all three.

Aerobics

Aerobic exercise is any exercise that temporarily increases your heart rate. How can you tell? By listening to your body (are you panting hard? Is your heart pounding? You've raised your heart rate) or by taking your own pulse (more on that in Chapter 9, "Life at the Gym"). Walking briskly, dancing, running, swimming, basketball, and even some types of yoga are aerobic. Aerobic exercise is great for strengthening the fitness of heart, lungs, respiratory system, and circulation. If you're interested in weight loss, it also burns calories.

Strength- and Muscle-Building

Strength- and muscle-building exercise works on increasing your muscle mass and strength, usually through free weights or machines at the gym.

For strength- and muscle-building exercise to make any difference, you need to do it at least twice a week. And you can't just go to your big brother's room and steal his barbells. Weight-lifting requires initial guidance from somebody who knows the ropes. You need to learn the correct positions and weight for your body. School P.E. teachers and coaches can help get you started, as can a gym pro (if you're doing the gym thang). There's more on this in Chapter 9.

Stretching

Stretching improves your range of motion and flexibility, and is good for your posture and your long-range alignment. Stretching also improves your circulation (because it raises your heart rate slightly). Got cold feet? Stretching helps. Stretching can also help you wake up in the morning on a foggy, groggy day. Dozing off in class? Stretch!

PHAT Fact

Stretch before any exercise, but start your exercise before stretching. Sound like a contradiction? Just get your blood moving for a few minutes by walking or dancing around (raise your body temperature a little), then stretch. It's more effective. Really.

Fitness on *Your* Schedule

So how do you fit it in? You don't have to become a jock; even a little more physical energy spent each day can make a difference in how you look and feel. Before you even commit to a small exercise program, you can make a big difference in your life by activating your life! The following suggestions don't take any more time (they might actually *give* you time):

✧ Turn off the TV.

✧ Walk up one flight and down two.

✧ Ride your bike. That's right, the one that's been sitting in the garage since your birthday last year. Dust it off, put on a helmet, and ride to school.

✧ Don't just sit there and gab—pace while you're on the phone.

✧ Walk instead of constantly bumming a ride (this isn't as grim as it sounds—walking is interesting!)

She Sez

"Aw, man, but TV is my *life*."

—Amy, 13

Set Moderate Goals

How much should you be exercising? The Centers for Disease Control recommend half an hour of moderately intense exercise every day. The *Health Fitness Instructor's Handbook* recommends 40 minutes three times a week as a fitness goal. But that doesn't mean you should start suddenly trying to find several hours a week to work that bod. Start slow, and start small. Half an hour a day is a *goal*. You want to look for a challenge—not get utterly wasted and exhausted.

Getting the Gear

For some people, getting the clothes and gear is half the fun of working out. On the other hand, the clothing has little to do with actually exercising. Here's the scoop—you don't have to bust the bank to work out. At least not at first. If you try an activity and love it, the investment in special sports clothes and gear makes more sense.

But what about things like bikes, balls, ice skates, skateboards, skis, and so on? Put your lips together and say the following three words after me:

✧ Rented

✧ Borrowed

✧ Used

Oh, and here's a good phrase:

✧ On sale

Get the picture? The idea is for you to start "moving your lovely body" as columnist Jon Carroll says. Don't let finances get in your way—be creative.

PHAT Fact

San Francisco Chronicle columnist Jon Carroll writes, "Here's the true fact about diets: They are not the most important thing in promoting weight loss .... You've got to move your lovely body."

Exercise Clothes

When it comes to exercising, comfort is everything. Some sports and activities (especially team sports, martial arts, and dance) might have particular gear, but usually sweats or shorts and T-shirts are good for beginners. Certain dance schools require more specific clothing (more on this in Chapter 9) as do some martial arts academies (and I'll go there in Chapter 12). But even specialty activities like these often let beginners wear basic clothes to start.

Holding It Up

You do need certain items, however. You need support for your feet and sometimes you need support for ... eh hem ... *other* parts of your body. (We'll do shoes in a moment.)

✧ **Support bras.** If your breasts are medium to large, or even if they are smaller and feeling tender, sports bras support while constricting the breast tissue; for this reason, it's really important to not wear a sports bra when you're not exercising.

✧ **Jocks and cups.** For some high-impact sports (like running), guys might be more comfortable wearing a jock strap for support. For contact sports, like football, you might also need a cup for protection. Your gym teacher or coach will let you know if you need one.

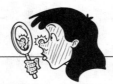

Beautiful? NOT!

Before you make a major gear investment, check out the activity for a while. The first class might be great, but do you really want to fill your closet with gear you've used only twice?

Shoe Shopping

You don't need fancy shoes for every activity, but it is important to protect your feet, especially for the higher-impact exercises like running, aerobics, tennis, basketball, and soccer.

What kind of a foot do you have? High-arched, "normal," or flat-footed? If you are clueless, wet the bottom of your bare foot and step onto a piece of colored construction paper. A flat foot shows a fat, complete footprint. A "normal" foot shows about half of an arch. A high-arched foot shows almost no arch between the heel and ball area.

Specialized Shoes

If you do a specific sport more than three times a week, you might need specific shoes for it. Here are some ways you can make sure that you get the right shoes for you.

✧ Feet tend to swell during exercise so you want shoes that aren't too small to begin with. Shop for shoes late in the afternoon after you've been on them all day. You want your feet to be at their largest.

✧ Wear the type of socks you plan to wear when you work out.

✧ Put on the shoes and wiggle your toes. You should be able to move those tootsies easily. Bend your foot in the shoe with your hand. It should be slightly flexible.

✧ Make sure your heel feels supported and doesn't rub up and down as you dash around the store.

He Sez

"I play sports 'cause I like to have fun. I get to see my friends that I wouldn't get to see otherwise. It's not that competitive, which is good, and it's also aerobic, but we don't really think about the aerobic part that way."

—Josh, age 14

Walking Shoes

Any comfortable pair of good, well-supported shoes are fine for a start (unless you're playing a court sport, where there might be certain requirements about color of your shoe soles so you don't mark up the floors). Ask for cross-trainers if you will be doing walking plus other activities, and be very clear when you tell the shoe salesperson what you need the shoes for. She or he will let you know if the cute shoes you like are appropriate.

High-Impact Shoes

For running and dance aerobics, you need shoes with padded heels that are higher than the soles and have a fitted heel cup. You're gonna be hopping up and down a lot, so protect your joints and bones! Running shoes tend to be lightweight, but unless you're a serious racer, avoid buying a shoe that's too lightweight. Aerobics classes and basketball require a lot of lateral movement (jumping), so look for a sneaker that comes up high in the back to keep your ankle from rolling over.

Tennis, Biking, Dancing, and So on Shoes

Don't mix your shoes. Shoes for tennis have side-to-side support that's missing in running shoes. Biking shoes are very stiff to help propel you down the road. Dance shoes depend on the type of dance you do—salsa, ballet, flamenco, tap, and so on. Talk to your teacher, talk to the shoe salesperson, and get the whole shoe story.

Nine Steps to Exercising Safely

Few sports are totally free of injury risk (except, for the most part, swimming). But you can keep yourself relatively injury-free by following these steps:

1. **Respect your body's messages.** If you feel pain, an abnormal heart beat, pressure in your chest, dizziness, or nausea, *stop!* If you can't get your energy back after exercise or are having trouble sleeping, *slow down!*

2. **Balance your muscles; balance your program.** Work major and minor muscle groups and combine aerobic exercise, stretching, and strength training to reach your goals without injury.

3. **Train by knowing—and pushing—the limits.** The key word is "pushing." You're not trying to "break through" your limit. Let your body get used to a level, and then push it a little more. Or as the old slogan goes, "Train, don't strain."

4. **Care for your feet.** Good shoes and good grooming (clip those nails! Watch for blisters!) will keep them healthy—and running (or walking) happily along.

5. **Keep the impact low.** Too much jouncing and bouncing is hard on your knees and other joints. If you do high-impact exercise, alternate it with low- or no-impact exercise.

6. **Use good form and learn proper technique.** You'll prevent injury and look hecka fine working out, too!

7. **Combine exercise with eating well and getting adequate rest.** Exercise alone does not make you healthy.

8. **Always warm up and cool down.** Warming up increases your body temperature, starts you sweating, prepares your heart and muscles for more activity, and increases the blood flow to your muscles. Cooling down keeps the blood flowing and helps minimize soreness by flushing waste products out of your muscles.

9. **Stay hydrated.** Keep drinking water. You lose fluid when you exercise, and it's easy to dry out. Always drink a glass of water before you start working out, and keep drinking all the way through.

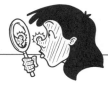

Beautiful? NOT!

Most sports injuries are to muscles rather than to tendons or bones. This is a good thing. Soft tissue tends to heal well—if you give it time! Don't try to push through an injury. If it hurts, stop!

The Least You Need to Know

✧ There's absolutely nothing more ravishingly gorgeous than a fit person.

✧ Exercise has a gazillion benefits. Plus, it's fun!

✧ Remember the three types of exercise: aerobic, strength- and weight-training, and stretching.

✧ Activate your life, start moderately, and listen to your body.

✧ You don't need fancy clothes to exercise in, but good, supportive shoes are vital.

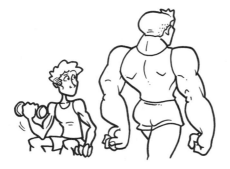

Chapter 9

Life at the Gym

In This Chapter

✧ How to choose a gym that's right for you

✧ Strength training tips and doin' the circuit

✧ All about aerobics classes

✧ Getting wet at the gym

✧ Personal trainers and over-training risks

I love going to the gym. I walk through the door and hear the clang of the machines, smell the sweat, see a collection of happy, sweaty people, and I breathe a sigh of relief. I'm here to work out. It's like a little vacation in my week—for the next hour or so I don't have to think about anything else, I just get to work my body. Gyms are, of course, incredibly popular with the older-than-teen set. But more and more, teens are joining gyms. Some are part of a family membership, but many just come to work out on their own.

This chapter is all about gyms—finding one and working out at one.

Choosing the Right Gym

Before you choose your gym, it's helpful to think about your overall goals. You need a gym where you can create a fitness program that will keep you motivated. Lisa Lewis, San Francisco fitness instructor and certified personal trainer, suggests that you consider a number of important elements before you plunk your money down someplace you might not enjoy.

Look for Convenience

Find a gym that's convenient to your home or your school, Lisa suggests, and I agree. Look, if it's hard to get there, you're not going to go. Oh, you might at first, but here comes the rain!

Check It Out, Baby!

Take a tour. Check out the facilities. Are the showers clean? (Gyms are regulated for safety and cleanliness—but some are just plain grody.)

What About the Pool?

If you're interested in swimming, ask when the lifeguards are on duty. Does the gym offer swim lessons? Are they included in your membership? It's a good idea to visit the pool during the busiest time and see how crowded the lanes are.

It's a Free Class! Take It!

Most gyms also offer an opportunity to take a few classes free of charge. Take them up on the offer!

Find out if the gym charges extra for classes (boo!) or if they're included (yeah!) in your monthly fee. Something else to remember about classes: They're not all the same from gym to gym (or even from instructor to instructor).

And if you're interested in classes, make sure they provide a wide variety. You might be into kickboxing now, but what happens if you want to switch to yoga in six months?

Are You Comfy Yet?

Ask yourself, "Is this environment comfortable for me?" What kind of people are working out? When you take a class, do you feel like the other students are all old fogies who you have nothing in common with or young bucks who are gonna stare at you and make you feel weird? You might not find a lot of teens at the gym—but you don't need to feel like a total geek for being there, either.

What about the staff? It might sound dumb, but it's really important that the staff be friendly. If you get a hard sell from the membership department, watch out (more on this in a moment).

Some gyms have segregated facilities or separate work-out areas for the men and for the women. Think about it: Do you like feeling scrutinized by the opposite sex? Do you care?

She Sez

"I was really nervous, 'cause I'm in really bad shape, and I thought everybody would be looking at me. But the lady who showed me around was really nice. I'm, like, the only one under 20 there sometimes, so I'm kind of like a mascot. It's fun."

—Kenya, age 16

Is It a Good Fit?

Ask yourself, "Does this gym provide the kinds of activities I like?" Some gyms are really focused toward weights. Others have a huge variety of aerobic classes and only a few machines. Make sure you check out more than one gym.

Cool Gym! Sign Me Up!

If you love what you see and experience and can imagine yourself there two to three times a week, working that body, it's time to talk with somebody in the membership department. Here's where things get sticky; you probably want to bring a parent along, just so you make sure you don't miss anything—it's easy to sign your life away. (If a parent will be paying for your membership with their charge card, or if the fees will come directly out of a parent's checking account, that person definitely needs to come with you.)

Your Options

Your options will vary from gym to gym, as will the price of membership. Here are some ideas of what a gym might offer:

✧ You will pay a monthly membership fee from around $50 a month to around $200 a month.

✧ You probably will also pay an initial enrollment fee—between $30 and thousands of dollars.

✧ Many gyms will give you a month-to-month option—if you ask. The fee might be a little more per month, but you don't have to give them your first-born baby if you leave.

The Agreement

At the end of the pitch, the salesperson is gonna put an agreement in front of you, hand you a pen, and wait for you to sign. Don't sign on the line yet—bring the agreement home and look at it!

At home, read all the fine print, and make sure you know what you're agreeing to. Are you contracting for five years? What happens when you go off to college? What's the cancellation policy? What happens if you're late on a payment?

Then figure out the nitty-gritty. How much will this really cost you? Will you get your money's worth? How often are you going to get to the gym? What does it break down to per visit? Is it worth it?

Pumpin' It—Strength Training

Wanna get strong? Wanna be built? Going to the gym for weights is definitely a pretty cool option. It used to be recommended that strength training was unwise for young teens. That's not true anymore, though you have to be very careful not to injure your growing body (yes, even if you've reached your full height).

One, Two Three, **Lift!**

If you follow certain guidelines, you should be fine and injury-free. You'll definitely benefit from the training (and not just socially from looking soooooo hot!).

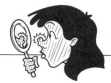

Beautiful? NOT!

Whoa! Don't do it! A study by the American Academy of Pediatrics showed that up to 3 percent of student athletes in middle school are using anabolic steroids. *Not safe!!* And definitely *not cool.*

✧ If you have any health problems (and this would probably include asthma), get an okay from a doctor first.

✧ Get instruction. Most gyms give a free orientation to the weight machines. Use it. You get your own program, and you're set.

✧ Especially with pumping iron, start small. Don't go proving anything—trying to bench-press your weight on the first go-round because your trying to show off will only demonstrate what somebody looks like writhing in agony on the ground with a set of ripped-out chest muscles (not pretty). Increase the weight (or resistance on the machine) gradually. And I mean *gradually!* You'll get there!

✧ Start slow. Begin with one set of 10 to 15 reps and adjust slowly. Aim for the eventual goal of one to three sets of 6 to 15 reps, two to three nonconsecutive days a week. (You don't want your weight days all in a row because your muscles need time to recover in between.)

✧ Become well-rounded (at least in your approach to weight training). Do a variety of weight-training exercises for both your upper and lower body, and focus on all the major muscle groups.

✧ Vary your program every few months, otherwise you're gonna get bored. And when you get bored, you're gonna quit.

✧ Don't rely just on weight training—it's only one aspect of a balanced exercise program.

✧ Make sure the machine fits you (or you fit the machine). Get somebody to check it for you.

He Sez

"The trainer at the gym was really cool. He didn't push me that hard on the machines, but he didn't let me slack, either. Now it's like, 'What's up, Bryan?'"

—Bryan, age 17

PHAT Fact

Focus on building your endurance with low resistance and high repetitions.

Circuit Training

You walk into the gym and there they are: the treadmill, the exercycle, the ski machine, the rowing machine, the Stair-Master, the climbing ergometer, plus all those Nautilus weight-training machines that make you feel like you're going to be strapped down and experimented on by aliens. You've got an hour to warm up, work out, shower, and boogie on out the door. Which fancy machine do you use? Why not all of them?

Circuit training is a great way to quickly work out your entire body. In circuit training, you move from one piece of equipment to another with a brief (30-second) rest period in between. You work out on each machine for anywhere between 1 and 10 minutes (that depends on the gym).

Some gyms have circuits specifically geared for strength training. Others are more aerobic-based. And still others are used primarily by classes instead of individuals.

Aerobics

Most full-service gyms offer aerobics classes of various kinds—spinning (done on stationary bikes), step aerobics, Cardio-kickboxing, and the more classic dance aerobics. Whatever type of exercise, the form is usually similar. An instructor (usually hopelessly fit and unbelievably attractive) leads the class through a warm-up period, a period of intense exercise designed to get your heart pumping at its optimum training rate (I'll help you calculate that rate in a split sec),

119

and a cool-down period. Sometimes the class includes strength training or body shaping at the end.

Your Training Heart Rate

Aerobic exercise only is effective when your heart works hard enough to reach your training heart rate—and stay there for at least 20 minutes. Figuring out your target heart rate takes just a few moments, but it's an essential piece of information if you're doing any aerobic exercise at all, to make sure you're working out effectively and safely.

To calculate your training heart rate, you need to know two things: your maximum heart rate and your resting pulse rate. Your maximum heart rate = 220 minus your age. So subtract your age from 220, and your maximum heart rate is: _____. (See, math is useful!)

Okay, now to find your resting pulse rate:

1. Place your index and middle fingers on the side of your neck, near your windpipe. Sometimes I actually slide them a little higher, under my jawbone.

2. Once you feel your pulse, put your eyes on the second hand of a clock.

3. Ready? Count the number of beats for six seconds.

4. Take that number and multiply it by 10. This is your resting heart rate. It's probably between 60 and 90. Your resting heart rate is: _____.

Okay, here we go: math time!

Minimum Target Heart Rate

To find your minimum training heart rate, take your maximum heart rate and subtract your resting heart rate.

Max. – Resting = _____

Take this number, and multiply it by .06.

_____ × .06 = _____

Now take *this* result and add the resting heart rate to it.

_____ + _____ (resting heart rate) =
_____ (minimum training rate)

Maximum Target Heart Rate

To find your maximum training heart rate, take your maximum heart rate and subtract your resting heart rate.

Max. – Resting = _____

Take this number, and multiply it by .08.

_____ × .08 = _____

Now take *this* result and add the resting heart rate to it.

_____ + _____ (resting heart rate) =
_____ (maximum training rate)

Working in the Zone

When you're working out aerobically, you're aiming to get your heart rate into the zone between the minimum and maximum training rate. If you're totally fit already, you can push the top end. If you're just getting started, you'll want to bounce along the bottom of the range for a while. Remember, once it's there, it needs to stay there for 20 minutes (or more) to do any good.

PHAT Fact

Drink your water! Dehydration makes you more sore.

How to Take Your Pulse During Exercise

How high is it? Should you take a break or keep on pushing? To figure it out, simply take your pulse for six seconds the same way you measured your resting heart rate and multiply that number by 10.

Whoa! It's Class Time

Aerobics classes provide a great way to get fit because all you have to do is show up—the instructor and the other students motivate you from there. They're also great because they're fun and, if you want them to be, a social time.

Spin It!

Spinning classes have nothing to do with those old fairy tales—you know—with the yarn, the spindle, the spinning wheel, and the 100 years of sleep. Nope, they're workouts—done to music and visualization—on stationary bikes. Spinning classes last 40 to 60 minutes. They're modeled after outdoor bicycle training sessions and try to replicate the experience of riding an outdoor bike.

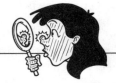

Beautiful? NOT!

You don't need to go fast to get the benefits of spinning. Going too fast is dangerous! Pace yourself. You're getting a workout at a slower speed.

The stationary bikes have a mechanism like a gear shift so you can regulate your own workout, and that's great, because it means you can train at your own speed, at your own rate. Plus you get those great thighs (see Chapter 10, "Outside

Exercise and Team Sports," for more on bicycling). This class is great for both beginners and experienced bicyclists. Start slow.

Dance It!

Dance aerobics classes come in a million different breeds. Every instructor selects her own music, and every instructor selects her own movements. In a dance aerobic class, you might be bopping to the blues or boogying to the Backstreet Boys and Britney. You might be slowly getting fit in a beginning class or competing with athletes in a super-high-powered, high-impact double session. What all classes have in common is warming up slow, doing a variety of easy dance steps over and over at a higher and higher pace, and then cooling down. All the while, the instructor is in the front of the room, modeling the steps so you can follow along. If you've never danced before, don't flip. I mean it when I say the steps are easy. They're easy enough that anybody can follow, even while panting!

PHAT Fact

Dance aerobics classes usually finish with stretching and/or weight work. Remember to do your own stretches later on as well.

Step It!

Step-aerobics classes have a number of similarities to dance aerobics. They're done to music, they warm up, work out, and cool down, and so on. Each student works out on a plastic portable step, moving up, down, over, and around it in a variety of steps. It's a great workout that focuses on your legs.

Step-aerobics classes were incredibly popular a few years ago. Now, the trendiest aerobics class has gotta be kickboxing.

Kick It!

Whether it's known as kickboxing, Cardio-kickboxing, or the Tae-Bo fitness system, it's hot. These aerobics classes combine martial arts moves with boxing punches, all set to music. Kickboxing is great fun and very good exercise, *if* it's done correctly. Be sure that you have a good instructor (and skip the home videos). You can easily injure the ligaments and joints in your back, shoulders, knees, hips, ankles, and elbows by overextending and by making too many harsh repetitious moves.

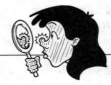

Beautiful? NOT!

How do you know if you're studying with a bad instructor? Bad ones push you too hard and don't seem to care about the risk of injury.

Wet It!

Water aerobics classes are completely nonimpact, which means that they are easy on the body. You do your dance steps in the water (no, this isn't water ballet—you're standing waist- to chest-deep as you exercise).

Lappin' It Up!

Swimming exercises all your large muscles and does it without stressing your body. It's also fun to glide through the water. Be prepared, though: Gyms usually have specific, strict rules about lane use in the lap pool. Often, you'll need to sign up in advance.

Getting Personal ... at the Gym

A personal trainer provides a variety of services, from setting you up with a weight program to—if you're Madonna or Demi Moore—spotting you for every lift and cheering and coaxing you through your exercise session. Most teens won't be hiring the services of a personal trainer on an on-going basis. Why not? Well, how does around $45 an hour sound? (And you can bet Madonna's personal trainer makes a lot more than that!)

Even so, you might still work with a personal trainer occasionally. A trainer can advise you on ...

✧ Healthy eating to improve your energy level.

✧ Weight management.

✧ Strength training.

✧ Setting up your training program.

✧ Calculating your heart rate, fitness, and goals.

✧ Providing on-going maintenance.

Your trainer should be a certified personal trainer. Most gyms either keep trainers on staff or have a pool of people they can recommend who are familiar with the gym and will come work with you there. Many gyms even give a free half hour with a trainer as part of the initiation packet!

PHAT Fact

When you're working out, you need water, water, water, and quick energy. For the energy, try an energy bar or a piece of fruit. And carry your own bottle of water from machine to machine to class to the sauna.

The Dangers of Over-Training

It's seductive to over-train. Watch out! Compulsive exercise can be part of an unhealthy body image. You're over-training if …

✧ You've lost energy and don't feel like working out.

✧ You're sleeping poorly at night but just can't keep your eyes open during algebra in the afternoon.

✧ You're not improving.

✧ Your morning resting pulse rate suddenly is higher.

✧ You keep adding extra workout sessions to your week.

✧ Your memory is going, and you're afraid you're coming down with a premature case of that aging disease, C.R.S. (Can't Remember Squat).

The Least You Need to Know

✧ Find a gym with the services you need, at a place where you feel comfortable.

✧ Review the membership agreement carefully. Some bite!

✧ For weight and strength training, get some advice about your program.

✧ An effective aerobics workout takes you to your target training heart rate zone and keeps you there for at least 20 minutes.

✧ Aerobics classes offer workouts to music for every taste, type, and level of fitness.

✧ A personal trainer can set up a program for you once or hold your hand through every workout.

✧ Avoid temptation! Don't over-train!

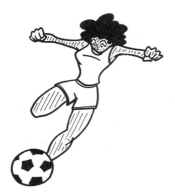

Chapter 10

Outside Exercise and Team Sports

In This Chapter

✧ Using your feet for fun and exercise

✧ The cold stuff—an intro to skiing and snowboarding

✧ Two-wheeling wonder—tips for beginning your bike program

✧ Joining a team

✧ Tips for staying safe outside

This chapter is an introduction to some of the basics of exercise on foot, on wheels, in the snow, and—with a group of others—on the field. What do they have in common? Well, these are all activities that are primarily done outside.

Of course, whole books are written on each of these subjects; this is just a start, like those yummy little spoonfuls of ice cream they give as samples at the ice cream parlor. Sample, savor, and decide which flavor scoops you'll try today.

PHAT Fact

Carbo-load! Carbs are the primary fuel source of energy in the body. The diet of a physically active person should consist of 60 percent to 65 percent carbohydrates. If you're truly athletic, this range of percentages goes up—to 65 to 70 percent carbohydrates.

Fun on Foot—Walking, Jogging, Running

Walking is the original—and some say, best—form of transportation. Walking as exercise ranks way up there in terms of fitness, plus it's free and you can do it anywhere in the world. Walking and running can be parts of your exercise program, or they can *be* your exercise program. Walking is also the first step on the way to running (remember that old slogan, "You gotta walk before you can run"?).

Walking the Walk—It's Not Strolling the Mall

Walking for exercise is not strolling, stopping for a bit, meandering some more, and so on. Walking for exercise is an aerobic activity, which means you need to get your heart rate up to your training rate (go back to Chapter 9, "Life at the Gym," for review!) and keep it there for at least 20 minutes. Walking for exercise means walking hard, and walking fast.

Power It Up!

You've seen those Mom-type women walking very, very quickly through the mall, water bottles in their hands, determined looks on their faces, sweaty headbands on their heads, and a really weird sort of stride. They're power walking, and yes, power walking looks kinda loony at first. It's actually really fun (you feel as if you're gliding across the earth). Power walking is walking—at the pace of a jog or run. You have to keep one foot on the ground at all times. If your knees hurt or you don't enjoy running, power walk it! (Just keep away from the headbands, and you'll be okay.)

Alternately, in jogging and running, you push yourself off the ground, and there's a little moment in each stride when you're actually airborne. Here's the interesting part: It takes the same energy and burns the same amount of calories to briskly walk or to run a mile—walking just takes longer.

Adding Accessories

To boost your exercise while walking, you might consider adding some elements.

So, What's a Jog? What's a Run?

In horses, there's a big difference between a trot and a gallop, but humans have two legs, not four—so there aren't that many ways we can move across the earth. In other words, jogging and running are really the same thing—running is just faster. Jogging also sounds like exercise, running sounds like a sport—your choice!

Gotta Run? Wanna Jog?

If you're making the shift from walking to running, do it slowly. The most common mistake people make is to start jogging at too fast a pace. Do the walk/jog thing for a while, until you've built up your stamina. Listen to your body.

From a jog to a run is a matter of degree—how fast feels comfortable? Running is pretty addictive. It feels great, and it's a great stress reliever. It's also a terrific way to challenge yourself. If you're running more than three times a week for more than a half hour at a time, you're probably running for more reasons than just aerobic exercise or losing weight. You're becoming a runner.

PHAT Fact

Consider saving up for some good quality sunglasses. They can help prevent squinting and road glare for runners and bikers, and snow blindness for skiers and snow boarders. Not to mention that they'll make you look like a pro.

What's your goal? Keep your training program gentle, and add on the miles gradually. If you're interested in running competitively, you'll need help from a running program or a private coach. (And, once you're in full training—for marathons or speed races—you'll have a variety of dietary needs that only your coach can help you with.) If you jump into heavy training too fast, you're risking injury. Listen to your body, and if you're tired, rest!

Snow Sports

The snow sports are ideal for people who love nature, and who love challenging themselves. If you're a speed demon, here's a place where the landing can be relatively soft. (I'll get into safety in a sec.)

There's a lot of tension between skiers and snowboarders, because even though the sports are similar, the people doing them tend to have different interests and certainly have different needs. You probably won't see both on the same slopes. Skiers face forward and shift from left to right to descend the hill. Snowboarders always face against or away from the mountain. They take bigger turns and go farther in each direction before making these turns. With these bigger zigs and zags down the mountain, there's a lot of risk of interfering with—or being interfered by—skiers.

Skiing

Skiing has always been the most popular winter recreational activity in the United States. Getting out in the snow is a blast; so is gliding over a snowy countryside, zooming down hills (the wind whooshing through your hair), and hanging out sipping hot chocolate afterward. Skiing is an international competitive sport; it's also great recreation. If you ski infrequently, be prepared for your legs and rear end to hurt the next day—unless you work out on a ski machine at the gym, you'll be using muscles you never knew you had.

It can be pretty costly to ski, and it can really add up if you do it a lot. You have to rent your boots and skis if you don't already own them, get out of the city and up to the mountains, and, once you're there, buy a lift ticket (the lift takes you up to the top of the slope so you can ski down). Unless you're lucky and local, you need to figure out where to stay, too. Cross country skiing is cheaper—you aren't paying for the resort.

What You'll Need

Here's a list of preliminary equipment you'll need for skiing:

- ✧ Boots
- ✧ Skis
- ✧ Poles

Buying all this gear will cost you hundreds and hundreds of dollars. Now don't flip out; it's way better to rent it daily or weekly. Even if you've stopped growing (and it's really hard to be sure when you're a teen), you probably haven't reached your adult weight. Skis are sized by weight and height. Because shoe size, weight, and height change so much as a teen, it's really not bright to buy equipment (unless you're already heading toward being a ski pro—in which case you don't need to read this section of the book at all!).

PHAT Fact

Rental skis come pre-fitted with bindings (the hardware that holds your boots to your skis and releases automatically when you fall) to help prevent serious injuries.

You can rent an equipment packet at any ski resort, which should be about $25 bucks a day (that's in California—your area might be different); or, before you head up the mountain, you can rent it at a sporting goods store for about half the cost. It's best to get your gear together before you go. Then, when you arrive, you can just buy your lift ticket (if you're going downhill), and hit the slopes early.

Snowboarding

Snowboarding has rapidly been overtaking skiing to become the best and coolest winter sport.

Snowboarding is a lot more expensive than skiing—it's also totally trendy. While your lift ticket should be about the same, equipment rental is much more. For instance, instead of getting a weekend equipment packet for $25 (the skiing price), you'll pay more like $45 for a snowboard packet, including your boots, bindings, and board.

Cold Weather, Warm Clothing

Skiing and snowboarding happen in the snow, and (duh) the snow is cold. You're also exposed to the wind and sun, and all this means that your clothes are pretty important.

Here's a basic list of winter sportswear must-haves:

- ❖ Long underwear. Cotton is good; silk or wool is better.
- ❖ A turtleneck, especially for those cold days.

✧ A sweater. (Go for the smoother ones—the fuzzy ones pick up snow. Snow melts. Then you're wet.)

✧ Pants. Jeans aren't great because they're stiff, and they're cotton, which will get you very cold when wet. Go for wool, nylon, or one of those great stretchy snow pant substances. Stretch pants may or may not look great on you, but they're the best for flexibility. They won't bag out.

✧ Socks! You'll need two pairs: a light pair next to the skin, and heavy wool or thermal socks on top. Make sure you wear them when you're getting your boots fitted.

✧ Hats keep your head warm, but it's more than that—a lot of your body heat is lost through your head. If you keep your head warm, your whole body stays warm.

✧ Hey, it's cold out there! Get yourself a good parka or fleece jacket.

✧ Sunglasses (for the glare)—they're necessary.

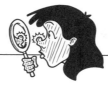

Beautiful? NOT!

For snow sports, wait until you're outside and booting up before putting on your socks. If you're inside, your feet will get hot and sweaty and you're gonna have damp socks. Damp socks equal cold feet. Cold feet equal grumpy you.

Getting Lifted

When you get to your resort (unless you're doing cross-country skiing) you're gonna have one more sticker shock when you go to buy your lift tickets. Here's where doing your homework helps—very often, supermarkets or various products will have advertising promotions to get you lift tickets at a reduced cost—if you buy ahead of time or bring a coupon. The regular cost of a lift ticket might be around $30, depending upon where you are. It's worth calling the ski resort in advance (yes, even if it's a long-distance call) to ask if they have any promotions going on.

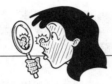

Beautiful? NOT!

Careful! Skiing is safe for beginners and gets more dangerous the more experienced you are. Beginners tend to go slow. Advanced skiers can get overconfident, over-tired, ski into trees, and become seriously damaged—or die.

Skiing and Snowboarding Safely

I hate to harp on it, but moving really quickly on one or a couple of little planks down a steep, icy hill is really dangerous. If you're hitting the slopes, take these safety measures:

✧ It's not very sexy, but wear a helmet, no matter how experienced you are. Most of the people killed on the slopes die of brain injuries (not to mention the ones who have to live as drooling vegetables!).

✧ If you're a beginner, take lessons from certified trainers on the easy slopes. Even a half-day lesson can be enough to start—it will be fairly cheap and a whole lot of fun.

✧ If you're intermediate, don't push it by skiing or snowboarding on advanced slopes! They're really scary and dangerous, and who knows who could be barreling down on you, expecting you to be able to zoom expertly out of the way …

✧ If you're experienced, watch out for slow-moving, less-experienced bozos (the ones just mentioned) and gauge your own fatigue. Accidents happen late in the day, and accidents happen when you're tired.

✧ Be especially careful if you're on a mixed-use slope—snowboarders and skiers often just don't mix.

✧ Moonlight and twilight are romantic—and often fatal—times to recreate in the snow. Aiaiaiaiahhhh! Look out for that tree!

Doin' It on Wheels—Bicycling

Bicycling is one of *my* favorite sports; it fits my solo spirit, plus it's exercise for a purpose (it gets you where you want to go). Biking provides great aerobic conditioning, thighs to die for, and great circulation. Bikers look great! Get into biking and your body will be a lean, mean, cyclin' machine. Biking is great for around-town transportation; it's also good for long distances. I've done a fair amount of touring, ridden with bike messengers in New York City, and even crossed France by myself—through the storms and against the mountain headwinds.

PHAT Fact

Biking burns about 500 calories an hour if you're going at 12 mph. In order for it to be aerobic, you have to go fast enough and far enough. Raise your heart rate to "training" level for at least 20 minutes per session.

Biking as a sport can be a true solo adventure, and it also can be a group activity. The great thing is that it's up to you.

He Sez

"Getting out on the road, the bike between my legs and nothing else around, is the best thing in the world. I forget about all my other stresses and just pump my body."

—Robert, age 17

Getting Going

First of all, you need a bike. Duh. But the one that's been in the garage since you were 10 might not be appropriate anymore. For one thing, it probably doesn't fit your body.

What Kind of Bike?

Off-road mountain bike or on-road traditional bike? For around town? Racing? Touring? You don't know what you need until you know what kind of bicycling you want to do. Biking is a science and a passion—and everybody has their own ideas about, for instance, the best length of chainstay for a touring bike.

Your Resource, the Local Bike Shop

Best solution? Go to a bike shop, and start asking questions. The people there know all there is to know … and this section can really only touch the surface. In general, here are some guidelines for choosing a ride-around-town bike:

✧ If you have an "average" body, one that's not particularly bigger on the top or the bottom, go for a bike with small, light wheels and a compact frame.

✧ If you're apple-shaped (bigger up top), balance might be an issue for you, and as a result, so will turning. When you go on your test ride, pay attention to the turns. Are you toppling over? (You don't want to be an apple turnover!)

✧ Pear alert! Those skinny bike seats can be a pain in the patootie if you tend to carry your weight down there. Ask for a comfortable seat and fully suspended wheels.

Once you have a bike that works with your body, you can start to ride. Biking is, as they say, like riding a bike. Your body never forgets how. If you learned when you were young, you'll have the basics down.

Ready to Ride

If you're getting into biking as a sport, plan to start gently, with two to three workouts a week (with rest days in between). As with any sport, listen to your body. Tired is great, total fatigue is too much.

PHAT Fact

An expensive bike can be fun—and expensive! You don't need to begin with the best. Yeah, it's fun to learn to drive using a Mazaratti, but you can learn just as well, get from point A to point B, and gain independence driving Dad's old Taurus.

Getting Serious

If you're serious about biking, you need to build your endurance. Serious riders often get into condition by riding—

hard—two hours a day for several weeks. If you're getting this fanatical, it's important to take care of your body by not working too hard. Always give yourself a rest day!

Organized Tours?

Biking is not necessarily a solitary activity. You can do it with a friend or friends, or in a larger group. Most communities organize bike tours. Some include people of all ages, others are geared just for teens and slightly older. Some rides are fairly short (30 miles or so), and some push you to do a full century (100 miles). If you want to try a tour, ask for recommendations at your local bike shop (or just look on their bulletin board). A group tour is possibly the best introduction to real riding.

PHAT Fact

Question: What do cyclists wear under their cycling shorts?

Answer: Nothing!!!

On-the-Road Biking Musts

If you're going more than a few blocks from your house, you need to think a little farther ahead.

- ✧ Always carry a patch kit and tire irons for patching flat tires—and know how to use them!

- ✧ Carry your cell phone if you have one, and be aware that it might not work in rural areas. What's your coverage?

- ✧ Don't forget the water! Water! Water!

✧ I believe in toe clips. From an exercise point of view, they makes sense: They reduce strain on your Achilles tendon and knee ligaments and tendons. More than that, they make your "stroke" more effective because you're not just putting force on the pedal going down, you're putting stress on the pedal coming up as well.

✧ Wear your helmet! (Yes, even for pedaling to the corner for a carton of milk.) My friend Ami was training for the AIDS ride on back country roads when she had an accident, landed on her face and lost five teeth and some jaw bone. Only her helmet kept her alive.

PHAT Fact

May all your flats be front ones, and may the wind be always at your back!

Team Work (Baseball, Softball, Football, Tennis, Soccer ...)

You might have been playing team sports since you were three feet tall, or you might be considering them for the first time. From soccer to baseball to football to lacrosse to field hockey, teens have always played outside sports. Some are available through your school athletic program (and that's how most teens are usually involved) and some through outside recreation leagues.

Teaming Up—It's a Blast!

Playing with a bunch of others is fun. You get to know people apart from the regular social grind of school, you gain a sense of comraderie and that sense of uniting for a common goal. People you never imagined being friends with (maybe they're into a totally different kind of music, a different scene) will surprise you by being loyal teammates. Playing on a team means you gain lasting relationships and have the chance to build experiences as well as skills.

It's not just about team spirit and hanging out with your buds, though. Team sports require an understanding of strategy and group dynamics. They challenge the mind, as well as the body.

What's the Commitment?

If you're doing a school sport, you're making a major time commitment. Practice might be every day after school, and possibly some evenings (especially at the junior varsity and varsity level). To play on a school team, you'll probably have to try out. Check with the coach of the sport to see what kind of skill level you need to join the team. Some coaches will work with athletes of all skill levels, while others require athletes to already be fairly skilled.

She Sez

"When I'm stressed and I go to soccer practice, it comes out. I play really, really hard; I take it out on the field and my teammates. If I have stress when I go, I let it all out on the field and it's good."

—Arden, age 13

Recreation department leagues usually don't require as much time commitment as school teams, but you might need to give up some weekend moments (well, hours, really). Sign up early! Because usually pretty much anybody can play, slots fill up fast.

Who's the Coach?

A huge part of your experience as part of a sports team will depend on the coach. The coach sets the tone of the team; the coach is the boss, the big brother or sister, the confidante, the supreme leader, the buddy, and the teacher all rolled up into one person with a clipboard and a whistle. It's worthwhile to know something about the coach before you get involved in the team sport.

PHAT Fact

Don't forget the water! Runners can lose more than two quarts of water in an hour. If you're getting headaches, amber or yellow urine, dizziness, or nausea, you might be dehydrated.

Outside Safety Do's and Don'ts

Exercising outside feels good. Instead of the loud whir and clanging of machines, the echoes of voices, and the view of a blank wall in front of you, you stretch and move and push your body through fresh air and birdsong. But working out outside does bring certain risks. Whatever your form of outside exercise, keep in mind the following safety tips:

- ✧ At night, exercise with others.

- ✧ Avoid deserted areas and listen to your intuition. Does it feel dangerous? Trust that feeling. Get out of there. Now.

✧ Protect yourself against the elements. Hats help to avoid sunstroke in the summer heat and, in the winter, keep out the chill. (In the winter, don't forget the other layers. Wear socks on the hands as mittens—you also can use them to wipe your runny nose!)

✧ Run against traffic.

✧ Bike on the side of the road (not in the middle) and go the direction of traffic.

✧ Yield the right of way to cars.

✧ Turn the walkman off. Yes, even on a very quiet street or in the woods! Walkmans are for treadmills and other boring inside exercise.

The Least You Need to Know

✧ Walking is a great—and free—form of exercise.

✧ A walk keeps one foot on the ground at all times. A run includes airborne moments.

✧ If you use walking accessories, make sure they're healthy and don't put a strain on your body.

✧ No matter what your exercise, go slow!

✧ Rent your ski and snowboarding equipment before you hit the mountains. You'll save money and time.

✧ Your local bike shop is the best resource for all biking questions.

✧ When considering team sports, ask yourself, "Who's the coach?"

✧ Always be conscious of safety risks including cars, awful people, and terrible weather.

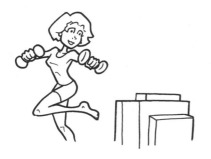

Chapter 11

Home Base—
Working Out
at Home

In This Chapter

✧ Your guide to stretching out in the living room

✧ Plug in, turn on, and work out with videotapes

✧ Exercise equipment and the "big machine"

✧ Everything you wanted to know about dumbbells (but were afraid to ask)

✧ Staying motivated at home

So, you don't like gyms, rec. centers, school locker rooms, muddy fields, or country roads? You have another option. Get fit without leaving your house or apartment!

You can add just a little exercise in the cracks of time between homework and dinner, or before bed. You can stretch on the rug while watching TV or do a quick set of push-ups to relieve stress before calling your crush on the phone or asking your parents for money. You can also undertake a serious get-fit program at home. This chapter discusses all of it. From stretching and warming up (for activities outside the house) to working up a sweat in the living room, this chapter is about exercising at home.

Your "Looking Great" Stretch

Stretching out your muscles is a reflex. Watch a baby sometime—Little Boo Boo wakes up from her nap. What does she do? Yawn and stretch. Stretching is an essential part of exercise, too. Regular stretching ...

- ✧ Helps make you flexible and limber by loosening your muscle tissue.
- ✧ Helps pump blood into your outer limbs.
- ✧ Increases your strength.
- ✧ Increases your recovery rate from exercise.
- ✧ Decreases your risk of injuring yourself during exercise.
- ✧ Helps keep you from getting sore after exercising.

You can stretch—informally—in bed in the morning before you climb out and face the day. You can also stretch more formally—with yoga exercises, dance stretches, or simple athletic stretches.

Everyday Stretching

Stretching every day will help you feel great. If you spend a few moments stretching every day, you won't need to stop and stretch before and after exercising.

For effective stretching ...

- ✧ Wear loose, nonbinding clothes (or no clothes at all).
- ✧ Before you begin any stretching (except for stretching in bed), walk or dance or jog for a few minutes to get the blood moving and raise your body temperature.
- ✧ Stretch slowly to where you feel slight tension. You might even feel a small amount of discomfort—but *not* pain.
- ✧ Don't bounce. Bouncing can tear your muscles. When you bounce, you risk over-stretching and injuring yourself.

✧ Hold each stretch 30 to 60 seconds (and never more than 90 seconds). Stop before it hurts.

✧ Do each stretch three times.

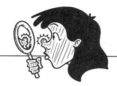

Beautiful? NOT!

If you stretch on a daily basis, you don't need to stretch right before or after exercising but you still need to warm up! Don't skip your warmup!

A Simple Stretch Series

Try these stretches! They'll get the blood flowing and the muscles lengthening. Find a clear (and clean) spot on the floor near a doorway, put on some comfortable threads, and get going!

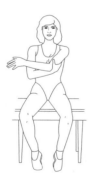
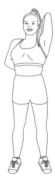

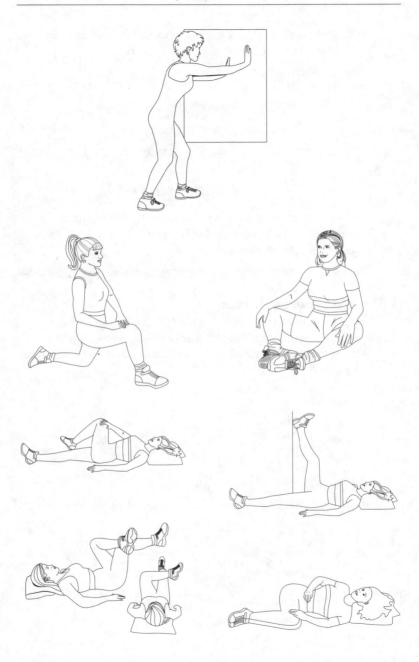

Video Trainer!

It's an easy solution—get on your sweats, plug in the video, forget about how stupid you might look if somebody walks in (that's the hardest part), and start exercising!

Your local video rental store probably has a wide selection of exercise videotapes from basic aerobic dance workouts, to kick boxing to the ones that focus on abs, buns, or inner thighs. Some are geared to older people, some to teens. Some feature celebrities. Some are almost soft porn, some are for beginners, and some are for serious athletes. Try them out before buying! Make sure that you love the music, that you can live with the trainer, and that you like the program.

It's important to keep in mind that nobody can correct your form when you exercise with a video (technology might be advanced, but it's not that advanced yet!), so it's important to keep an extra-close eye on yourself—perhaps by working out in front of a mirror. If something hurts or feels weird, stop doing it!

Home Exercise Equipment

So you want to work out and you don't want to go to a gym. Maybe you love the idea of listening to your music—loud— or watching TV while you get fit. It's certainly possible—anything you can do at the gym you can do at home, if you've got enough money, room, and self-motivation. Stationary bikes, rowing machines, bench presses .... Home exercise equipment is far more than a dusty treadmill in a corner (although we'll talk about that in a sec). You can even buy an all-in-one machine where you can work every major muscle group in your body.

The Dust Collector

Many people buy home exercise equipment, use it for a brief time, and then give up on it. They lose interest, they lose motivation, they feel lonely working out alone at home or— and this is a reason many people don't understand—the

147

equipment doesn't work as well as it did at the gym. (It's cheaper and not made as well!) No matter what the reason, most home exercise equipment does end up blocking doorways and serving as a great place to drape your old clothes.

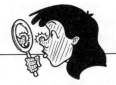

Beautiful? NOT!

An exercise machine controls how fast you go. Yes, of course you can adjust it! But it's driving you, not the reverse. Be very careful to use machines at a pace that is comfortable for your body, or you risk injuring yourself.

High End vs. Low End

Home exercise equipment starts out reasonably priced (a couple of hundred dollars for a good bench and dumbbell system) and goes up to thousands and thousands for a high-end, multi-tasking machine that the whole family can work out on at once—the warranty is forever, and there's an espresso machine powered by the automatic ratcheting device (okay, just kidding about that part). So, which do you go for? Quality or price? I suggest limiting the features, but buying as much quality as you can afford.

Quality counts here. The gauge steel (that's the thickness of the metal used to build the machine—you want it pretty thick), the welds, the workmanship, the comfort ... you get what you pay for. Here are some other things to consider when you're buying exercise equipment from a store:

❖ The warranty. Cheaper equipment is under warranty for 90 days. The "good stuff" might have a lifetime warranty on the frame, three to five years on parts, and one year on labor.

✧ What kind of servicing is offered by the store you're buying it from?

✧ Will they deliver your equipment, or is it you and your buds out there with a borrowed truck?

✧ Will someone from the store come out to set it up for you? (This is well worth paying for—all those screws, adjustments, headaches ... unless you enjoy that sort of torture. No judgment! Some people do.)

He Sez

Eric Thompson, a manager of Omni Fitness Equipment Specialists in Oakland, California, says that the average time people use a piece of exercise equipment bought at a garage sale is "Oh, about a week or two, maximum." Then it becomes *your* dust collector and clothes rack.

Why Drop So Much Cheddar?

Okay, this stuff is expensive. Not just a little expensive; I've bought cars—good cars that actually drive for years and don't look like complete junkers—for less than some of the current home gym systems.

When is it worth it? If ...

✧ You like to work out on a certain machine (like a treadmill or stationary bike).

✧ You belong to a gym and you pay all this money every month but all you do is work out on that same machine.

✧ You are self-motivated enough to work out in your own home (while the refrigerator bleats, "Open me!" and your phone keeps ringing).

And ...

✧ You have the room and the money.

Then ...

✧ Getting an exercise machine for your house might be worth it.

The Big Machine

Got an extra $1,000? Got an extra $10,000? You can have a gym in your own home. Known as the "Home Gym" or "Universal Gym," these are single-unit machines that let you do everything except wash the dishes.

Basically, they are weight machines that enable you to work every major muscle group (and probably a lot of minor ones, too).

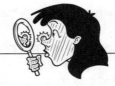

Beautiful? NOT!

That treadmill you use at the gym costs between $6 and $10 kilo-clams. The treadmill you might buy at a low-end discount equipment store might cost $500. Don't expect them to feel—or perform—the same.

Walking to Nowhere, Cycling to Oblivion

When the weather stinks and you want to continue your outdoor walking, running, or biking, it's great to have your own exercise equipment. And, some people prefer working out inside to outside anyway. If you're a runner, running on a treadmill is low impact. Remember to work at a pace that suits your body.

Many people use exercise machines as a way to warm up, before stretching, and before moving on to something else (like running or playing a sport). You can use your home machine for this purpose, too.

The Complete Idiot's Guide to Dumbbells

The simplest—and cheapest—weight workout is right there in your bedroom with dumbbells. You have three basic choices: dumbbells, adjustable dumbbells, and nesting dumbbells.

She Sez

"When I began to run, everybody was looking at me. I'd rather work out at home, where nobody sees me jiggling."

—Norma, age 16

Dumbbell Delight

These come in a variety of styles: hexagon, neoprene, rubber hexagon, and chrome (listed from cheapest to most expensive). Dumbbells usually are sold by the pound. How much you want to spend depends on you and what purpose you use them for. You can spend hundreds of dollars getting two of each size (one for each hand). Or you can start small, and add the sizes you need as you go.

✧ **Hexagon.** Your standard dumbbell. Hexagon dumbbells cost around 70¢ a pound (they might vary in your area). These are metal dumbbells—perfectly fine for lifting and other exercises. You might consider gloves with these (they can be rough on the hands).

✧ **Neoprene.** These dumbbells are coated in smooth, nice-feeling plastic, and come in a variety of cool colors. Neoprene dumbbells cost almost twice as much as standard hexagon dumbbells.

✧ **Rubber hexagon.** Like regular hexagon, but rubberized. Advantage? They do less damage when dropped and are easier on the hands. Disadvantage? More than twice as expensive!

✧ **Chrome.** The Cadillac of dumbbells, chrome dumbbells cost around $2.00 a pound (remember that you need two of each size). Smooth, rust proof, sleek. Chrome dumbbells only go up to 50 pounds.

PHAT Fact

When you're buying dumbbells, buy only up to a weight you can comfortably lift. Add on as you go!

Make Room for the Dumbbells!

Dumbbells take up space. You can get a rack, but that costs more money, and while a rack takes care of keeping things tidier, it doesn't solve the space problem. It might even add to the space problem! If you live in a small space, you're better off with a different system.

Adjustable Dumbbell Handles and Plates

This might be your cheapest option. You buy a couple of chrome handles (they cost less than $15 each) and a bunch of weight plates (at about 50¢ a pound). The plates screw on to the handles, and you're ready to rock 'n' roll, dude. But remember, you need to buy them in sets of four—two for each dumbbell. The main disadvantage of this system is that they are bulky, and you might end up changing the weight plates several times during your workout.

Nesting Dumbbells

This is the ultimate system when you have a small workout space or live in a small apartment. If you know you want a system with weights from 5 to 45 pounds (or 3 to 21 pounds, or 5 to 100 pounds), you can buy a nesting weight system. All the weights nest together in two cubes. You select the amount of weight you want to lift, use the pins to lock that amount of weight in, and away you go. The initial outlay is a little more (small sets run around $120 and bigger sets run $250 and up), but buying all those weights as individual dumbbells would cost a lot more.

A Bench Is Not a Bench

A bench is about the simplest piece of exercise equipment you can buy, right? So why not go for something cheap? Well, it's a myth. A bench is not a bench ... some benches are far better. What should you look for in a weight lifting bench?

- ✦ A flat/incline/decline adjustable bench (This gives you the biggest range of motion.)
- ✦ Strength and workmanship
- ✦ Padding (Too wide and it will limit your range of motion, too narrow and you'll topple off.)

✧ Ease of adjustment (You don't want to be wrestling the bench instead of working out.)

✧ Extras (What positions does it go to? Does it have any add-ons?)

Some Dumbbell Exercises

There are oh-so-many things you can do with dumbbells! These exercises are just a start.

Shoulders

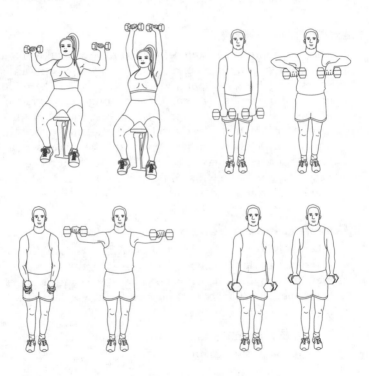

Chest

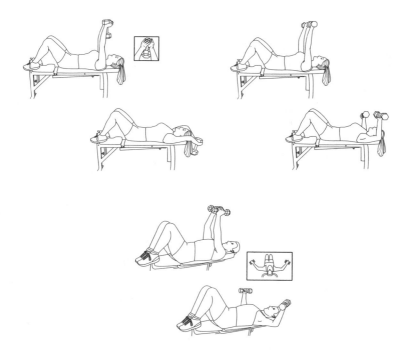

Biceps

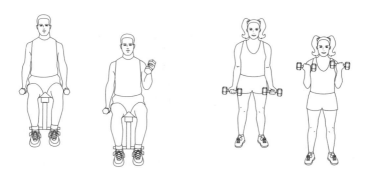

Triceps

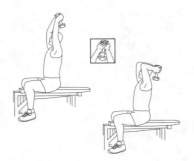

Legs

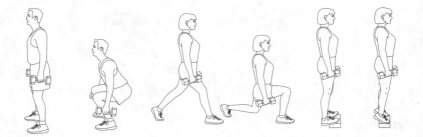

PHAT Fact

Girlz, you're not weight training 'cause you don't like that bulky look, right? Start lifting! A good weight training program will build your strength without bulking you up. Use low resistance and high reps to define and tone.

Working Out at Home

Whether it's stretching, running, cycling, pumping iron, or using an exercise video, working out at home can be fun ... and it can be mind-numbingly boring. Exercise shouldn't be a drag. It can feel great (yes, even while you're doing it). Make the experience fun for yourself.

Movin' to Music

Here's an advantage to working out at home—you get to play whatever music you want, and you don't have to wear headphones to do it. Well, at least if the adults in the house agree. Moving your body to music feels awesome and serves as a great motivating force.

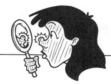

Beautiful? NOT!

Don't hold your breath during an exercise. It's dangerous, and might cause you to get dizzy or black out! Exhale when you lift, inhale on the return.

Treading to the TV, Moving with Mags

If you're on a treadmill or a bike, you might want to watch TV or read a magazine at the same time as you walk or pedal. It can make the time whiz by (since you have no scenery whizzing by).

Nobody Said You Had to Be Alone!

What's wrong with having friends over to work out with you? Or even (if you can bear seeing them in their torn-up sweats) your long-suffering parents?

Motivating Yourself

It can be really hard to motivate yourself at home. If you're a member of a gym and you make yourself show up, you'll probably feel motivated enough to complete your workout. If you're on a school team, the coach is there to get you going. At home, alone, it's only you. If you review your long- and short-term goals (go back to Chapter 2, "Improvement!? You're Not Out to Lunch," or check out what you've been writing in your "Looking Great" Journal), you might get a new hit of motivated energy.

Then again, motivation might not be an issue for you. You go!

The Least You Need to Know

✧ Stretching increases flexibility, improves strength, and works best if you do it every day.

✧ Try out a lot of videos before buying one.

✧ Home exercise machines are usually not as good as the ones in the gym—unless you spend a boodle of money.

✧ Dumbbells and a bench are a fairly inexpensive option for your home workout.

158

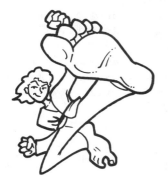

Chapter 12

Martial Arts—Far Eastern–Style Fitness

In This Chapter

✧ Why learn to fight?

✧ Styles and secrets of the martial arts

✧ Choosing the right dojo for you

✧ Getting belted—moving up in rank

Interested in kicking out, punching solidly, making a single move and watching your opponent fly over your head and onto the floor? Want to walk fearlessly through your neighborhood, alert, aware, and confident? Martial arts can be tremendously empowering, and they're a great deal of fun.

Kickin' It with Martial Arts?

Martial arts are sports, exercises, and fighting techniques. More than that, they are philosophies. They all stress self-defense and a holistic approach to life. Studying a martial art works out your body and mind, gets you fit, and gives you a great sense of confidence. You'll also be able to defend yourself if you ever get into a tight spot. Martial arts schools also tend to be close communities—if you're studying at a dojo (martial arts school), you might gain a new community of friends.

Learning to Deal with Intensity

Studying martial arts gives you a sense of how to remain calm in the middle of wild physical activity, and this translates to the rest of your life. Martial arts students swear up, down, and sideways that their sense of overall serenity improves so that, whether it's fists, feet, chairs, homework, tests, or screaming parents flying at their heads, they can assess the situation and calmly step aside. This makes martial arts a great stress buster.

PHAT Fact

Girls and women sometimes feel fear about their physical safety, and martial arts can help. Even a pro has vulnerabilities, but a female with martial arts training can better identify dangerous situations, avoid them, and cope when physically threatened.

So What Are the Martial Arts?

High kicks, Bruce Lee, "Way of the Dragon," slow-moving T'ai Chi, breaking boards and bricks, wise masters in white loose clothing with black belts—martial arts are all these and far more. The martial arts are fighting arts and sports that largely came from the Far East. Some are done mostly for health and spiritual development, some stress fighting techniques for self-defense or even warfare, and some are primarily sports.

All martial arts combine a sense of discipline in a fairly formal atmosphere, but this sense of dignity and structure can be reassuring and stress-relieving. All the arts aim to develop integrity, perseverance, courtesy, self-control, and indomitable spirit. And none of this takes away from a prime quality of martial arts training—it's fun!

The martial arts are divided into two styles: hard and soft. Hard styles (like karate) stress kicks, chops, punches, and blocks. You'll get a lot of muscle and strength training but will have to work harder to get an aerobic workout. Soft styles (like Aikido) use the opponent's own energy to throw him or her off balance (the goal is to defuse the situation physically without hurting anybody). Soft-style martial arts tend to be very aerobic and help increase your balance and strength.

He Sez

"I studied for three years. I did it with a whole group of friends, and it was really fun. Doing martial arts was really cool. In a way it kind of opened me up to different things, different activities."

—Josh, age 14

Martial arts are also divided into "grappling" (joint lock) and "striking" (hitting and kicking) styles. All the styles are valuable—it's up to you and your preferences (as well as what's available in your area).

Karate

Karate means "empty hands" and was developed in Okinawa in the fifteenth century but now is practiced (in a variety of forms) in China, Japan, and just about everywhere else. Practitioners use their bare feet and hands to strike, punch, and sweep their opponents (this is not a grappling-style martial art), though it also incorporates weapons. Karate is more aggressive than, for instance, Aikido. Karate takes years to master—it's a very challenging art—but you gain some skills quickly. Most karate schools incorporate competition and tournaments as part of the curriculum or activities.

Jujitsu

Jujitsu was developed in Japan and is known as the "science of softness." It's the root of Judo and Aikido (see the later sections). When you study Jujitsu, you learn to turn your opponent's force against him and use leverage to attack him. Jujitsu is a soft, grappling, fighting art but it also includes punches and kicks when they're needed.

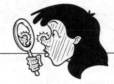

Beautiful? NOT!

Don't mistake "soft" martial arts for sweet, gentle, mushy styles. Soft styles can be the toughest—Jujitsu, a soft, grappling style, is used by armed forces for hand-to-hand combat.

Judo

Judo was developed from Jujitsu in the late eighteenth century as a sport for Japanese schools and colleges, rather than as a fighting art. Judo is basically Jujitsu with the dangerous elements removed. The more aggressive kicks and holds are removed, and sweeping, unbalancing throws added. Judo is called the "way of gentleness." If you're studying Judo, you'll gain balance, flexibility, speed, and accuracy, and practice remaining alert with a serene and calm mind. It's a soft, grappling-style, defensive martial art.

Aikido

Aikido, meaning "the way of harmony with universal energy," also comes from Jujitsu. It was developed in 1931—a baby compared to some of the other martial arts! Aikido is a purely defensive, soft-style martial art that stresses finding harmony in the relationship between the mind, the body, and the participant's outlook on life. Aikido uses quick movements to turn the opponent's force back on himself—there's no punching and no kicking at all. Aikido artists evade and shift to avoid blows or other attacks and then move suddenly to control, and often floor, an opponent. Watching Aikido practitioners sparring is very beautiful and quite amazing.

PHAT Fact

Aikido participants, who practice a "grappling" art, have more injuries than participants in the various "striking" arts.

Tae Kwon Do

Tae kwon do is probably the most popular martial art in the United States. A Korean art known for its high and jumping kicks and powerful punches, tae kwon do is a hard- and striking-style martial art known as "the art of hand and foot fighting." Participants focus on striking high above their heads (the original purpose was for foot soldiers to attack soldiers on horseback). Board-breaking is important in this style as a technique to demonstrate mental discipline and power. Tae kwon do also stresses the important balance between nature, body, and mind.

Kung Fu

Kung fu (also known as Wushu) means "skill achieved over time through practice," and truly "getting" kung fu requires a lifetime of study. Better start now! If you watch old Bruce Lee movies, you can get a sense of the art. It incorporates elements of both hard and soft, but basically, it's a striking, rather than a grappling, style.

T'ai Chi

The "supreme, ultimate fist," this slow-moving, connected-movement style is one of the oldest martial arts in the world. T'ai Chi focuses on harmony with others and with life. It's more philosophical and spiritual than many other martial arts. The patterned movements are designed to clear the mind, reduce tension, and focus the energy. Participants learn to yield so that an attacker defeats himself with the force of his own attack.

PHAT Fact

Testing for a black belt generally costs $100 to $200.

Capoeira

This Brazilian martial art is done to music—so it looks like dance—a deadly dance indeed. Capoeira means "rooster." It was developed by African slaves brought to Brazil by the Portuguese. It's highly acrobatic, as combatants face each other in the Roda, the center of a circle made of other dancing participants, to compete with kicks, handstands, and posturing like roosters fighting while musicians play. Capoeira is very demanding.

Thai, Indonesian, and More Martial Arts

Various other cultures practice martial arts of different types. Muay Thai is the kickboxing tradition of Thailand. Ninjutsu (you've heard of Ninjas, right?) is a Japanese practice that includes information gathering, hand-to-hand combat, wilderness survival, and stealth. Ninjas get so in touch with the environment that they can seem to disappear. Other cultures also have martial arts, including the Philippines.

PHAT Fact

One of the worst things about working out regularly is getting a small injury or a cold and *boom*, you're out of action for days. In martial arts, you can always practice in a limited fashion.

Doing It at the Dojo

Practicing a martial art means perfecting certain movements by repeating them over and over again—and these will be different for each style. There are also a variety of other activities you'll do as part of your training.

Learning the Forms

The basic martial arts techniques include punches, kicks, or throws (depending on the style). Besides practicing these, you'll spend time doing *kata* (sometimes known as *hyung*)—or forms—which are sets of movements that a martial artist memorizes and practices. Forms let you put the techniques together in a flow; they emphasize balance and grace. Most of the time you do your forms alone, though some styles have partner forms.

Sparring

Besides practicing your techniques and working on your forms, you'll also be sparring. In step sparring, partners take turns attacking each other, with the defender blocking and then stopping the attacker. A freestyle sparring situation more closely resembles a real fight, with both partners attacking and defending at the same time. Freestyle is more advanced (obviously!) and usually requires safety equipment.

Bricks and Boards

In many styles—particularly the Korean styles like tae kwon do—participants break bricks and boards with their bare hands. Why? First of all, it's better to demonstrate your power on some*thing* rather than some*body*. It's also a confidence builder. If you can snap a board (which is about an inch thick) you know you can snap somebody's rib. It's also a way to discipline the mind (you're up there and thinking, "Yow! This is gonna hurt!" and then you gain the strength to overcome the pain and do it anyway). And finally, if you do a technique wrong, the board won't break. The instructor can see clearly whether you've got the technique nailed or not.

The Loud "Haii Yahhh!!" (or: What Is Chi?)

Martial arts schools focus on cultivating *chi* (in Chinese, or *ki*, in Japanese) in each participant. The chi is "the life force," and is centered in the abdomen and controlled through breathing. (Work with breathing exercises is called "chi kung.")

PHAT Fact

Martial arts are about strength, confidence, conditioning, and power. But studying martial arts shouldn't feel like a drag or a duty. Martial arts should be fun!

Martial artists believe that the correct use of chi can make a person more powerful than physical strength—it's the ability to focus all your determination and energy on one task or target. Martial artists focus and express their chi through their shout (called a *kiai* or a *kihop*).

That Amazing Sense of Calm

Martial artists spend a lot of time learning to stay calm and focused. When you're calm and detached, you're less concerned about physical harm, and you're able to think and react more clearly and quickly. This calm quality is vital to create the kind of intense focus needed for martial arts. As part of martial arts training, many schools offer—and encourage—meditation training.

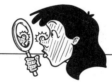

Beautiful? NOT!

Don't forget to warm up and cool down with serious stretches when doing any martial art. This will help prevent injuries!

You Gotta Have Heart

Technique, strength, calm, and focus can only take the martial artist so far. The true martial artist also has heart and spirit. A deep belief in your abilities, combined with understanding and compassion, will help you succeed as a martial artist.

Martial Arts—Not Just for Guys

Fighting and martial arts traditionally are dominated by men, but things are changing profoundly, and lots of women study martial arts. You should know that …

✧ Not all schools totally encourage women—so find a female-friendly school that does (and lots and lots do!). Note that "female-friendly" doesn't mean wimpy. It just means that nobody cares that you're a girl, and they respect you for who you are.

✧ You might face a little attitude problem from one or two Neanderthal brutes. Let the head instructor know what you're facing.

✧ Try not to let sexism get to you—and if it is, and if it isn't resolvable, find another place to train! (My friend Saill, who studies Aikido and is the head student in her dojo says about girls and women studying martial arts, "You *will* encounter bullies/misogynists/creeps just like everywhere else on the planet—I think it's a small but ubiquitous fraction of all guys. Changing dojos if only 10 percent of the guys are that way is senseless, and it'll probably be worse somewhere else. Sticking with it and learning to stay calm and focused around that energy could be extremely valuable.")

Finding a Dojo

Finding a dojo (school) is a serious thing—think about it before running down and signing up. Your experience will vary so widely from style to style and from dojo to dojo. A dojo represents a community, a philosophy, and a way of life.

Before you commit to a dojo, here are a number of items to consider (with thanks to the book *Martial Arts for Women*, by Jennifer Lawler):

✧ **Location.** Find out what schools are available near you. Think about how close they are—how will you get there?

✧ **Martial arts style.** Since martial arts styles vary so widely, you might need to do more research about the different styles.

✧ **School.** How long has the school been around? What's its reputation?

✧ **Classes.** What kinds of classes do they teach, at what levels, and at what times? Do they work for you and your schedule?

✧ **Motivation.** Are you seeking a black belt or just a way to get fit? Do you want to compete (and does the school emphasize or support competition)?

✧ **Instruction.** Watch a class and ask questions later. What do you think of the instructors? What are their qualifications? How do they dispense discipline?

✧ **Facility.** Is the school clean? Are there enough mirrors, and are the mats in good shape? How's the lighting? Are the bathrooms filthy or clean?

✧ **Size and class makeup.** How big are the classes? How big is the school? What size do you like? Are there classes just for teens, or do teens work out with the adults? Do you like that?

✧ **Contact.** Find out the amount of contact for the particular style and school (and think about how comfortable—or uncomfortable—contact makes you feel).

✧ **Cost.** How much does it cost, and how do they charge (by the week, month, or year)? Do you get unlimited classes for that amount? How much does testing (to advance to the next belt rank) cost?

Getting Belted

As you move through your training, you'll periodically test to reach a higher rank. Your improvement and your skills will be marked by the color of the belt you wear. Most martial arts styles begin with a white belt. Belt colors include yellow, green, orange, blue, purple, brown, red, and, of course, black.

Rankings can feel very important, and preparing for a ranking test can be a lot of work.

The Least You Need to Know

✧ Martial arts are sports, exercises, fighting techniques, philosophies, and a great way to get fit.

✧ Martial arts come in a variety of styles: "hard" or "soft," "striking" or "grappling."

✧ As part of your training, you'll learn fight techniques, forms, how to spar, and, in some styles and schools, work with weapons such as staffs and swords.

✧ Choosing (or re-choosing) a dojo might be the most important decision in your martial arts training.

✧ Martial artists move up in rank through a series of tests—and ranking is shown by the color of the belt you wear.

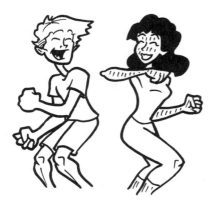

Chapter 13

Dance—Finding Your Rhythm

In This Chapter

✧ What dancing can do for you

✧ Details on dance styles

✧ How to choose a class and a studio

✧ What it's really like to be a dance student

Why dance? Why not!? It's a natural form of expression; it's fun and very creative; it gives you strong body awareness; builds strength, flexibility, and coordination; increases your self-esteem and improves your health. Dance is based on the love of movement. You might say that dance is the finest form of exercise (and if you said that, I wouldn't disagree!).

Everybody's a Dancer

Dancing, like singing, is natural. Kids hear music and move their bodies to it before they can walk. It's a primitive instinct, an emotion that moves your body when you listen to music. Tell the truth: Haven't you ever danced wildly around your bedroom, alone?

There's dance in every culture in the world. People use ritual dance in their religious practices, they dance socially with—and for—each other, and they perform dance for audiences in theatrical settings.

When you study dance, you might end up performing, or you might not. Whether your goal in dance is theatrical, social, or both, dance can be a valid exercise program and a creative and ritual way to express yourself. But most of all, dancing is fun.

But Then You Get Embarrassed!

Dance might start out as a response to a primitive emotion, but something sad and odd happens to a lot of people as they grow older—they become self-conscious. And after a while, only "dancers" dance anything more complicated than an occasional free-form boogie. People are embarrassed about dancing.

PHAT Fact

It's a crime that dance is considered only a high art form in our culture; it is a widespread misconception that only "dancers" can dance.

A Special Note for the Guys

A male ballet dancer friend of mine used to be called "Twinkle Toes" by the guys in the machine shop where he worked. He answered by: 1) Kicking his steel-toed boot exactly right up to—but not into—the ear of one co-worker, and 2) Saying, "Hey, 9 out of 10 people who study dance are women. I spend my off hours working with—and watching—beautiful women moving their bodies while wearing very little clothing." His colleagues switched from teasing to admiration and envy.

As a male taking dance, you'll build your body and your strength and, if you're serious about dance, you'll have a far easier time becoming a professional. Men are like gold in the dance world. They get the roles, they get the attention, and, if they want them, they get the girls.

Dance Improves Your Body

There are zillions of dance styles, but they all have several characteristics in common:

- ✧ **They're aerobic.** Dance speeds up your heart and makes you sweat.

- ✧ **They build strength.** Dance requires power and strength. Some dance forms (like ballet) are more physically challenging than others.

- ✧ **They keep you limber.** Dance stretches your muscles and keeps you flexible.

- ✧ **They're artistic.** Dance is an art form, a way to express emotion.

Dozens of Dances

There's a dance style for everybody, and every body.

Some of the dance classes currently offered near where I live include Apache, African-Brazilian, African Modern, Afro-Cuban Folk, Afro-Haitian, Afro-Samba, Balinese, Ballet, Ballroom, Belly Dance (tribal style), Bop, Brazilian, Break dance, Butoh, Can Can, Carolina Shag, ChaCha, Clogging, Congolese, Country and Western (including line dancing), Flamenco, Folk, Funk/Street Funk, Guinean, Hawaiian, Hip Hop, Hustle and Disco, Foxtrot, Improvisational, Javanese, Jazz, Jitterbug, Kathak (North Indian), Lindy, Modern, Modern Jive, Odissi (East Indian classical dance), Polynesian,

Paso Doble, Round dance, Rumba, Sacred dance, Salsa, Salsa-Rueda, Samba, Square dance, Swing, Tango, Tap, Tarantella, Thai, Vogue and New Vogue, West African—and this is just the beginning.

I don't have room here to describe all the dances and dance forms, but here are some brief descriptions to get you started.

Ballet Basics

What do circus trapeze artists, ice skaters, football players, and gymnasts have in common? All are likely to study ballet to improve their form and performance. Ballet is, in many ways, the classic Western form of movement. It's not all tutus and stiff formal movements!

What makes ballet ballet? Toe shoes, dancers moving in a grand manner, leaps and turns that dazzle—these are what we usually think of as ballet. But ballet can also be more in-formal, and sometimes, downright weird. Ballet is ballet when it is theatrical dancing—with costumes, lights, and sets—performed by dancers who've been trained in classical ballet movements.

She Sez

"Do you know about boys taking ballet? My teacher told me that football players take it. Professional football players."

—Annie, age 12

Finding a Ballet Class

Ballet can be hard on your joints—if taught poorly. It's very important to study ballet with a good teacher at a good studio. How will you know? Ask questions. The care the teacher takes in answering your questions will tell a lot about the teacher and the studio. Here are some questions to put to the teacher:

✧ How long have you been teaching?

✧ How large are your classes? (Smaller is better—you get more personal attention.)

✧ What's your teaching philosophy and approach to ballet?

✧ Are you more geared toward performance or enjoyment?

✧ How do you work to prevent injury?

PHAT Fact

Classical ballet movements are described with French terminology, words like: plié, relevé, bettement, and rond de jambe. These translate into basic descriptions: bending, raised, beating, and "round of the leg," for example.

Modern Dance Mystique

Modern dance began about 100 years ago as a backlash to the rigidity of ballet. Lois Fuller, Isadora Duncan, and others felt that dance should celebrate the body. Modern dance is based on more "human" movement. It's usually done barefoot, the heels maintain more contact with the floor, and the torso moves in ways that traditional ballet teachers might consider shocking.

In modern dance, bodies don't all have to look alike! Modern dance troupes include dancers with every body shape and every body size. Modern dance provides a great deal of flexibility and tremendous creativity—which might be why older ballet dancers often shift to modern dance.

Just because modern dance is flexible and creative doesn't mean it can't be challenging. It is!

PHAT Fact

Isadora Duncan is considered the mother of modern dance. Her students, young girls who danced in white Grecian robes with flower garlands in their hair, were known as the … (hang on to your lunch) "Isadorables."

Jazz Joy

Jazz dance is a kind of modern dance set to pop music. Most people think of jazz dance as the kind of dance you'll see in Broadway musicals such as *Cats* or *A Chorus Line*—flashy, intricate, combining the loose torso of modern dance with the spins and leaps of ballet and the glitz and flash of show business. Jazz dance varies so widely from teacher to teacher and from studio to studio that it's hard to characterize it … just know that you'll have a blast, you'll work your body hard, and—depending on the teacher—you might challenge your mind trying to remember all those steps!

Jazz dance classes tend to be filled with teens. Why not? You gotta study before you move to New York to become a star!

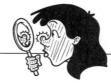

Beautiful? NOT!

A dancer does not have to—should not have to—be skinny as a skeleton. Too many professional dancers become anorexic trying to match some impossible ideal. Plenty of dance forms allow real bodies. Focus on one of those—or fight to change the system. Don't hurt yourself.

World Dance—Impossible to Categorize!

So-called "world dances" are folk and traditional dances from around the world. The movements, the rituals, and the traditions vary so widely that they are completely impossible to categorize. There are "folk dances"—dance styles that have been created—over time—by the people of a particular culture to be performed and done by everybody, and "traditional" dances—dance styles that might, for instance, have been used to entertain royalty.

You might choose to study a world dance form because it reflects your culture or your roots, or because you think the music sounds great, or because you love the movements.

✧ Formal Southeast Asian temple dances are rooted in a completely different sense of aesthetics than, for instance, ballet (which really is a Western "world" dance).

✧ Traditional East Indian dance is highly disciplined, each movement carefully choreographed.

✧ African dance is as varied as the continent; from the intricate, earth-oriented foot movements of the Yoruba dancers in Nigeria to the upright, high-stamping movements of the military Zulu dancers of South Africa, and everything in between.

177

✧ Flamenco dance is steeped in Spanish gypsy culture and closely tied to the soulful singing. Live singers often accompany dance classes.

Urban Dance

One recently developed dance form that comes from America's cities is called "urban dance"—it's developed by ordinary dancers rather than professionals and reflects contemporary urban culture. Urban dance includes Hip Hop, Break dance, Stomp, and Funk. It's all about attitude, baby!

Tap Tap Tapping

Tap dance, like jazz dance, is another "show" dance. Dancers use their feet as percussion instruments as they dance. Tap dance started as an American slave dance—the taps were actually a form of sending messages through walls and behind the masters' backs. Tap dance got really square for a while, but it's back with a vengeance as the coolest thing in town.

Partner Dances—Swing, Ballroom, Salsa, Disco ...

Partner dances are largely "social" dances, although they often have a performance aspect to them. They're dances done—duh—with a partner.

✧ **Swing it!** You're probably aware of the big swing dance craze that happened a few years ago. Swing is still hot—jitterbugging to the big band beat ...

✧ **Latin dancing.** Most Latin dances (Tango, Salsa, Samba, Merengue, Rumba, Paso Doble, and so on) are done in pairs. They can be easy (one lesson and you're groovin' all night) and they can be incredibly athletic and complex. Most of all, like all partner dances, they're a blast!

✧ **Ballroom, Baby.** Ballroom dance is mostly a social dance, although ballroom competitions definitely lend it a "sport" aspect. You might think that ballroom dance is just for your grandparents. It's not. If you want to learn to ballroom dance, though, make sure to find a studio where the average age is 20, not 60.

Building Your Confidence

Trying a new dance form or a new studio? Take a beginners' class. Even professional dancers regularly take beginners' classes. It's a way to focus on technique without putting competitive stress on the situation.

When you leap into an intermediate or advanced class at a new studio—even if you've been studying somewhere else—you risk stressing yourself out. Start slow, take it easy, and have fun.

Choosing a Dance Class

What kind of class should you take? Try a few! Most classes don't require an initial commitment—you can take a sample class or two without signing up for a series (more on this in a moment). But if you want to hedge your bets and narrow the field, there are some things you should think about.

PHAT Fact

Dance gets you long, lean, limber muscles. It's a great choice of exercise if (like me) your legs tend to be short and thick.

The Dance Itself—Ya Gotta Love It

Do you like the way the dance looks when it's done right? If you hate disco, then studying the Hustle isn't a great idea. If you adore the Tango (even if your friends think you're a nut), consider trying a lesson or two. How will you know what you like? Watch them! Besides finding music videos on TV, go to the library and check out their dance video section. Look for dance videos put out by … The Kirov Ballet (*Sleeping Beauty*), Alvin Ailey, The New York City Ballet, Merce Cunningham, and whatever else you see that looks cool.

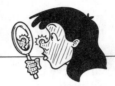

Beautiful? NOT!

Don't ever cheat on your warm up! More than almost any other form of exercise, dance requires warming up and stretching before you begin. It's way too easy to get injured—protect yourself!

Serious, or Fooling Around?

Dance classes—no matter what the dance or dance style, are divided into two basic types: classes where most students are there to relieve stress and have fun, and classes where most students truly focus on their technique. The first is a more so-cial dance class; the second, geared toward "serious" dancers, aims at preparing students for performance.

You might begin with one approach or intent (either one). Over time, you might switch your approach—and that's fine!

Boogie to the Beat

What kind of music is identified with the dance style? The bigger, broader dance forms such as ballet (no, it's not all sugar plum music), modern, and jazz use all sorts of music so you can't really know in advance what the teacher will use, but specific dances such as Salsa, Rumba, and Flamenco are closely identified with specific musical styles.

It's Social, So Who Are the Students?

What kind of people take a particular dance class? It's worth checking it out. If you love Swing dance, but all the people in the class are over 40, you might want to try the Hip Hop class instead.

On the other hand, groovin' with the old folks might be to your advantage—their bodies don't learn as fast—anywhere near as fast—as your body does. If you're intimidated by the Broadway-bound chicks and hunks who study at the local jazz studio, start with the old folks' class. You'll be the best and most limber in the class ... and that will build your confidence.

A Good Dance Teacher Is Positive!

Not all dance teachers are wonderful. Not all wonderful dancers make good teachers. You can—and should—be selective about who is working with your body. A good dance teacher ...

✧ Knows the dance style inside and out.

✧ Knows the best way to teach it to students.

✧ Loves teaching, and isn't just teaching to make a living so she can continue taking classes herself.

✧ Understands the risks to the human body and takes steps to minimize the risk of injury.

✧ Is kind, compassionate, and teaches through positive encouragement and specific, guided criticism rather than through harsh and negative critiques.

A good dance teacher also knows how to create an atmosphere of fun, enjoyment, kindness, and motivation inside the dance studio.

PHAT Fact

You have the right to not be abused or mocked by your dance teacher! Find a teacher who teaches through encouragement. They're out there—and you deserve it.

The Dirty Details on Dance Studios

Wanna dance? You can take dance classes at the gym sometimes, but generally you need to go to a private dance studio. Some studios are very formal and only teach a particular form of dance. Some are run by a specific dance company. Other studios rent out space or hire various dance teachers who teach different styles.

Look in the Yellow Pages under "Dance Studios" and start calling around. Ask for a brochure to be mailed to you—it's free, and it's what they like to do!

Money, Honey!

Dance can be an investment, but if you plan it right, your parents won't be out on the street begging for food just because you want to dance ... actually, it's not that bad. Most studios have several payment options:

✧ You can pay for one class at a time ($6 to $15, depending on where you live). This is the best option at first, while you're shopping around.

✧ You can buy a series card for a certain number of classes. This is where you start getting a financial break.

✧ Some studios have a monthly pass—you pay a lump sum and can come to as many classes as you want during that month. This is the best option for serious dance junkies.

✧ If you have any skills or want to help out, many studios will trade labor (answering phones, sweeping the studio, writing brochures) for classes. This is the best option if you're short on money but long on time. It's also a great option if you're really into the scene at a particular studio. You get to know everybody!

He Sez

"You're not getting me into those tights things."

—Morgan, age 16

What's a Dance Class Like?

People who've never danced are often surprised at how little dancing occurs in most performance-oriented dance classes. A classic ballet, modern, or jazz class generally follows the same pattern: You begin with a warm-up and stretching session on the studio floor to increase your flexibility. Then there's a session at the bar or on the floor where you work specifically on techniques and steps. Finally, students try out their technique by moving in dance combinations across the floor. If your class is working on a specific dance, here's where you work on that, too. Before you know it, bingo, class is over! You're hot, sweaty, and feeling great!

Classes in other dance forms might vary—but usually the pattern is the same: warm-up, technique, dance.

The Dancer's Attitude

Dancing is more than just learning steps and moving your body to music. It's an attitude—using your body to celebrate, express, and reflect emotion. Part of the dancer attitude is a respect for the human body and what it can do. It can look ethereal and otherworldly, leaping and spinning in ballet. It can elicit lust and sensual longing in the sexy, sultry Tango.

As part of this respect for the body's power, a dancer or dance student learns to be kind to the body—to nurture it, keep it from injury, and feed it well. A dancer needs strength—and strength means good nutrition, sleeping well, being aware of your own limitations to limit injury, and generally taking care of yourself.

The Least You Need to Know

✧ Dancing is a primitive instinct, and every culture has its dances and its dancers.

✧ Dance differs widely in style, music, and mood. Shop around!

✧ Figure out if the class you want to take is geared toward performance or enjoyment. Either is fine, but know what you're getting.

✧ You have the right to a positive, professional dance teacher.

✧ Ask about payment options. There are lots of ways to pay for dance classes.

✧ Treat your body with respect.

Part 5

Looking Good— from the Outside In

It's not all food and exercise, you know. Looking great is about the other stuff, too—your hair, your skin, your clothes, and most of all, your 'tude.

This section deals with the outside parts of looking great: dealing with zits, doing your toes, finding your own, personal style (and affording it!). And I ask you ... have you ever seen another book that tells you the nitty gritty details of how to shave your legs? You saw it here first, Baby!

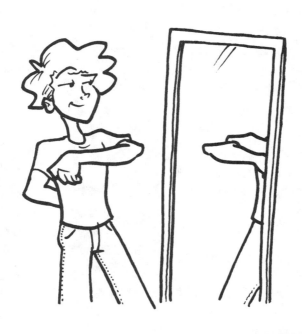

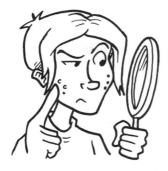

Chapter 14

The Skin You're In

In This Chapter

- ✧ Zit quiz! What really causes those breakouts
- ✧ Cleaning and treating your face
- ✧ Deadly skin sins: sun, smoking, sleep dep, alcohol, and stress
- ✧ Dealing with body hair—tips on taking it off

You know that it's what's on the inside that really counts, but it's your outside that shows—and face it, it's hard to feel great about yourself when your face is one large eruption. Skin's one of those things you don't think much about—unless it's giving you problems.

The Skin, Your Biggest Organ

What is skin? Your skin is the biggest single part of you, even though it's only about .08 inch thick on most of your body. Skin is made up of two layers: the epidermis on the top, which forms the tough outer layer that few germs can get

through, and the dermis below, which contains nerve end-
ings, blood vessels, hair roots, and sweat and sebaceous
glands. Until you're twenty-five or so, your skin is elastic. It
stretches and grows with you. Then wrinkles and creases start
to appear and your skin loosens—it doesn't bounce back as
easily as it once did.

PHAT Fact

Did you know that your skin is always shedding? In one
minute, you might lose up to 40,000 skin cells. They're re-
placed by new cells, pushing up from the bottom of the
epidermis.

Zit Quiz!

Okay, pop quiz: true or false? What (or who) is to blame for
that zit?

1. Chocolate, French fries, and more chocolate

2. Male hormones stimulating overly productive oil
   glands into overactivity

3. Your parents and grandparents

Answers:

1. **False.** Grease and chocolate don't go hand in hand
   with zits. For most people, unless they're truly allergic,
   it's not a 1+1 equation—Chocolate + You = Zits. Most
   doctors say there's little direct relationship between
   what you eat and pimples. (Of course, if you aren't
   eating well, your body is stressed, and when you're
   stressed, you tend to break out ... so you do the math!)

2. **True.** Your skin acts as a barrier against injury and disease. Natural oils, called sebum ("see-bum") coming from the sebaceous glands, coat the surface of your skin. They keep your skin flexible, and prevent water from seeping into your body. When you're a teen, you have an influx of androgen hormones (see Chapter 17, "Attack of the Hormones!"). These hormones stimulate extra sebum production, especially in what is known as the T-zone, which covers the forehead and runs down the nose and chin. Sometimes all this extra sebum clogs up a pore. Then the pore gets inflamed and ruptures— and voilà, a zit!

3. **True, too.** Skin—and its tendency to break out—is an inherited thing. It runs in the family. Here's something you can genuinely blame your parents for (though it's really not their fault!).

So what can you do? Other than not being born into your family, there's not a tremendous amount you can do about your tendency toward pimples. All's not lost—there's lots you can do to treat your skin. More on that coming up.

What Is a Zit, Anyway?

Zits, breakouts, and acne are a few words people use for the four kinds of eruptions that can happen to your skin. Specifically:

✧ **Blackheads.** The pore gets clogged up but stays open. The top surface gets dark, and you have a blackhead.

✧ **Pimples.** The pore gets clogged up and closes. It begins to bulge from the skin, and you have a pimple.

✧ **Whiteheads.** Bacteria gets into a pore. It infects the oil gland. It gets red and inflamed with yellowish pus and bulges from the skin, and you have a whitehead.

✧ **Cysts.** If you squeeze or pop your blackheads, pimples, or whiteheads, you can force oil and bacteria deeper into the dermis which can form large, painful cysts. If you squeeze a cyst, it can rupture and scar!

Your Skin: Care and Feeding

Your skin is your largest organ, and even when it's not totally broken out, it needs your love, care, and attention. Skin lecture alert: This is not your mother's skin! Normal adult skin has a pH value of 5.5. For teens, the ph is higher—more "basic" (that's all that sebum in action). As you might remember from your teacher Mr. Longyawner, droning on in science class, "acid" is at one end of the spectrum, "base" the other. The more "basic" the skin, the easier it is for bacteria to develop, leading to breakouts. What does this mean for you? Well, it might mean yet one more thing in your busy schedule—you gotta wash your face.

Skin care experts recommend that teens wash their faces at least a couple of times a day to clear the skin of extra oil, bacteria, and dead skin cells, and to rebalance the pH value.

How to Wash Your Face

Carefully! Splash warm water on your face, and, using a mild liquid facial cleanser and your fingers, cleanse carefully with an upward, circular motion. Don't …

 ✦ Pull at the delicate areas around your eyes and throat.

 ✦ Use soap, harsh detergent, astringents, or scrubs.

 ✦ No scrubbing, no rubbing! Scrubbing with a washcloth actually can create acne.

The idea is to *gently* exfoliate your skin while removing the dirt, sweat, and extra oil. ("Exfoliation." It sounds like leaves falling off the trees in Autumn. In the world of skin care, it means the removal of the invisible layer of dead cells that builds up on your skin.) Now rinse gently. Blot your face dry with a clean towel (don't rub!).

After You Wash, Tone It!

Many skin care experts recommend "sealing" the skin with a toner. The type of toner you use should depend on your skin type (and we'll discuss that in a moment). Toner tends to dry the skin, so you need to moisturize and replenish the skin.

PHAT Fact

Try a moisturizer that also contains sunscreen. You'll get your sun protection without the extra hassle of buying—and applying—a separate product.

... and Moisturize!

After you tone, use moisturizers to hydrate the skin and re-store the balance. Once again, the type of moisturizer you should use depends upon *your* skin.

The type of skin cleanser, moisturizer, and toner you need will depend on the type of skin you have. You might need to care for different parts of your face in different ways.

Skin Type	What Does *That* Mean?
Normal	"Normal" skin is neither dry nor oily. It's just right! Alas, not too many of us have "normal" skin. (Maybe they should call it "ideal" skin instead!) Your cleanser should be a mild product, your toner should be mild and alcohol-free, and you should use a light lotion to keep your skin hydrated.
Oily	If you have oily skin, your whole complexion shines from your overactive sebaceous glands. Your pores often clog up, leading to ZITS! Your cleanser should be oil-free, your toner should keep oil under control without drying, and your moisturizer (yes, you need one!) should be oil-free, yet still replenish the moisture you lose from dry air and soap.

Skin Type	What Does *That* Mean?
Dry	Dry skin is caused by under-productive oil glands. Your skin is dull, sometimes flaky, and your face feels tight when you open your mouth. You need a cleanser that softens and soothes the skin, a gentle, alcohol-free toner, and a thick, rich cream to replenish and retain skin moisture.
Combination	This type is most common for teens. The T-zone is oily and the cheek and eye areas are dry. You need to use a cleanser that is safe for all skin types, an oil-free toner for the T-zone plus an alcohol-free version for the rest of your face, and an emollient-rich moisturizer for the non–T-zone areas (your T-zone might not need moisturizing).

Breakout!

The best fight against zits is prevention—and prevention of bigger problems. Dealing with skin issues is sometimes more a matter of what you *don't* do than what you *do* do:

✧ Don't scrub! Scrubbing can help inflame matters.

✧ Don't touch that face! Keep your hands away from your face as much as possible to avoid spreading germs.

✧ Don't use dirty tools. If you use makeup, remember to wash your tools regularly (more on this in Chapter 17).

✧ Don't let your hair down. Get your hair off your face as much as possible. Bangs and droopy hair can transfer hair oil onto your face and cause breakouts.

✧ Don't get dehydrated. Drinking water helps flush out impurities and rehydrate the skin.

"Don't Pop" and Other Zit Remedies

Once you have zits, don't pick at them! It's a terrible temptation, but I urge you to resist. When you squeeze, tease, pick, pop, or even touch your pimples, you push oil and bacteria deeper into the skin. You can cause small but permanent scars on your face. If you have a pimple, you can take some of the redness out by applying an overnight drying agent. If you've got a cyst, apply a warm compress for a minute followed by Benzoyl Peroxide (see the following).

Over-the-Counter Medications

Over-the-counter zit medications usually contain some of these ingredients:

✧ **Benzoyl Peroxide.** Ye Olde Zit remedy. It helps the body loosen clogged pores and slough off dead cells, it kills bacteria, and it slows the production of oil. It also is a drying and peeling agent, so if your skin is dry, don't use products that contain it.

✧ **Alpha-hydroxy acids.** AHAs come from milk, sugarcane, and other fruits. They are good for mild acne and fine facial lines.

PHAT Fact

Your facial skin and your body skin have different qualities and needs—you need to treat them as different entities! That means no body lotion on the face! (It's likely to make you break out.)

What the Doctor Sez

If your skin gets bad enough, you might find yourself at a dermatologist. Aside from being educated on how to wash your face, you might be prescribed medications such as these:

- ❖ **Retin-A.** This is a topical cream you apply on your face. Retin-A makes the skin thinner and more sensitive to sun. It can irritate and cause peeling and scaling.

- ❖ **Accutane.** This oral medication is prescribed for severe cases of acne. It can be very effective, but it's very strong and very drying. People who use it often complain of dry lips, nose, and eyes. You'll need to use moisturizers and lip balms while on it. Accutane can have serious side effects, including liver damage, and it's been associated with birth defects, so you MUST NOT get pregnant while using it.

PHAT Fact

What you eat matters! While diet doesn't cause acne, it does cause beautiful skin. Eating fresh, nutritious foods will make your skin glow!

Skin Killers

To keep your skin looking great, you'll have to be conscious of the effects your behavior has on your skin. Your skin is like a mirror. It reflects where you take it (to the beach, to the pool), what you feed it (water and veggies or alcohol and cigarettes), how late you keep it up at night, and how much stress you're under. Yes, abusing your skin is a way to look older … if you want to look wrinkled and sallow. Be nice to your skin. Once the damage is done, it's almost impossible to repair.

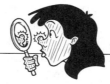

Beautiful? NOT!

If you have a mole that changes color, a new mole that appears suddenly, a bump that oozes or bleeds, or a "blurry" mole, see a doctor immediately! Melanoma (skin cancer) can be fatal but is curable if caught early enough.

Sun Protection

Sun is a skin killer, and sometimes a people killer, too. Long-term excessive exposure to the sun ages the skin prematurely, causing that not-so-lovely "early prune" look. Sunburns and frequent tans are a direct cause of skin cancer; every year, the sun causes one million new cases of skin cancer. With the thinning ozone, this number is going up! We're not talking old folks here—most damaging exposure occurs before the age of 20. To protect your skin ...

✧ Wear sunscreen on a regular basis, not just when you're going to the beach to fry. Use one that protects against both UVA and UVB rays with a sun protection factor (spf) of at least 15 (all of this information is on the package).

✧ Try to put on your sunscreen at least 20 minutes before you go out.

✧ If you're swimming, use a waterproof sunscreen.

✧ Reapply your sunscreen every few hours—even on cloudy days.

✧ If you're really fair, go for the lovely white linen look—the hat, the woven clothing, the shades—and shade. You're truly susceptible to sunburn (and skin cancer). Avoid the peak sun hours of 10 A.M. to 4 P.M.

✧ Yes! Dark-skinned people need sunscreen, too. Yes, yes, yes! While you might not easily sunburn, you're still exposed to cancer-causing rays. Very black skin provides some protection—equivalent to 15 spf sunscreen, or 45 minutes of protection.

Killer Smoke

The Surgeon General's labels on cigarettes stress only the truly evil things cigarettes do to the inside of your body: cancer (lung, throat, mouth, esophageal, pancreatic, kidney, bladder, and cervical); fatal heart disease; emphysema; peptic ulcers; and so on. The labels don't stress the wrinkles and yellow teeth and fingers that show up sooner. Smokers simply don't look as great as nonsmokers.

Sleep Matters!

Teens need lots of sleep! Rest shows up in your skin. Lack of sleep affects your skin's tone, firmness, and clarity. Staying up late too often will start showing up in how your skin looks, as well as in how dragged out you feel.

PHAT Fact

Up too late staring into cyberspace? To soothe puffy eyes, dip eye pads in chamomile tea and place over your eyes for five minutes. Looking raccoon-like? Try thin slices of raw potato over your eyes to remove dark under-eye circles.

Alcohol: Aging and Acne

Aside from the other risks of beer, wine, and booze (addiction, overdoses, car accidents, liver damage, sexual impotence, and so on), alcohol can devastate your skin, causing wrinkling and breakouts. (Whoa, pimples and wrinkles at the same time!) Drinking alcohol seriously dehydrates your skin cells. Excessive drinking also can cause vitamin deficiencies, which show up in your skin as well.

Stress Stresses

Stress and anxiety often lead to breakouts because they cause the adrenal glands to make more androgens, the hormones that stimulate extra sebum production in the skin. There's a whole chapter on stress later on in the book.

Body Hair—Busting the Fuzz

When we talk about skin, we have to talk about what's on it—hair—and talk about how to get rid of the parts you don't want. You furry thing! Depending upon your cultural upbringing and where in the world you live, hair can either be a good or a not-so-desirable thing. In general, we seem to like it on our heads, and less so on other places.

What you choose to do with your own body hair is your decision, based on what makes *you* feel comfortable: to shave it, pluck it, wax it, depilitate it, or let it alone to grow freely.

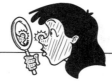

Beautiful? NOT!

Removing hair can make your skin sensitive to the sun. Always wait a day before going into the sun.

Shave It Off!

Shaving is one of the easiest and cheapest ways to remove unwanted fuzz. For guys, beginning to shave your face on a regular basis is a rite of passage. While guys usually only shave their faces (about 20 percent of men also remove back hair), girls often shave other parts of their bodies: legs, underarms, and sometimes crotch hair. To stay fuzz-free, you'll need to shave at least once or twice a week.

When you shave, you're using a razor to cut the hair off your body, right down at the skin level. Since you're not doing anything to the root of the hair, the follicle keeps pushing up new growth. You need to shave frequently, and, once you've begun shaving, the hair starts coming back thicker and more nubby. If you're a girl, never shave your forearms or your face—those are places you do not want stubble!

Here are some tips for shaving:

❖ **Lubricate!** Shaving creams and gels protect your skin from nicks and cuts and help you get a closer shave.

❖ **Go easy!** Always shave against the grain. And you shouldn't need to press down to get a smooth shave. Disposable razors should be disposed of every five to seven shaves.

❖ **Specialize.** A wide-handled razor is best for legs (gives you more control around those tricky ankles and backs of knees), a triple razor system (with replaceable heads) is heavier than disposables, and might be easier to work with.

❖ **Do it in the shower.** Hot water helps open your pores. Dry shaving is hard on your skin; you'll end up with red, itchy bumps (razor burn).

Pluck It Off!

For tidying eyebrows and stray chin hairs, plucking with a tweezer can be a solution.

✧ **Soften up!** Showering before plucking, or steaming your face with a warm, wet washcloth can help open pores and follicles, leading to a less-painful plucking experience.

✧ **Pluck in the right direction.** Always pluck in the direction of hair growth—you want to glide the hair out of the follicle, not break it off inside.

Melt It Off—Depilatories

Depilatories dissolve hair just below the surface of the skin, leaving silky smoothness. It's not permanent; you'll need to use depilatories once every week or 10 days to stay hair-free. Depilatories are best for fine hair and hard-to-reach areas like your bikini line. Never use it on course, kinky hair.

✧ Always test a small area first. Some people have allergic sensitivities to the chemicals in depilatories. If your skin gets red, swollen, or itchy, find another method.

✧ Get wet. Shower or take a warm bath before you depilatate. Warm water softens the hair. Dry completely.

✧ Slather it on—but DON'T RUB! Leave a thick layer on for four to eight minutes (read the label for exact instructions) and then check a small patch by wiping away the depilatory. If the hair's still there, wait another couple of minutes. But no more than 10, tops.

✧ Rinse it all off without rubbing. You can use a warm, wet washcloth to gently remove the last traces.

✧ Still hairy? Wait 24 hours before you remove any leftover hairs still hanging around.

✧ Soothe it. If the skin looks red or feels irritated, try a thin layer of 1 percent hydrocortisone cream to reduce irritation.

Rip-p-p-p!!!! The Joys of Waxing

Waxing is a form of hair removal that pulls hair out from the root. Waxing lasts two to four weeks, depending upon hair thickness. For those who regularly remove hair from the body, that's a whole lot of time spent *not* shaving, bleaching, plucking, or smelling chemical depilatory. Note: You've gotta be hairy to begin. Hair has to be at least ³/₈-inch long so the wax can get a good grab.

What about the Ouch Factor—Does it hurt? Yeah, a bit. But really, no more than ripping off a Band-aid. It's over in a split second, and you get used to it. Your skin also gets less sensitive the more you do it. A tip for soothing skin after waxing: Salons recommend antibacterial gel for the first day after an area has been waxed. Try not to use soap on the area for 24 hours.

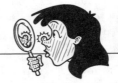

Beautiful? NOT!

If you use Retin-A, Accutane, or similar products, DO NOT WAX! These products make the skin very thin and sensitive. Waxing can burn or rip the skin right off your body.

Waxing Yourself

You can wax some parts of your body yourself, such as legs and bikini line. For underarms and eyebrows, waxing can be tricky. Try another technique, or leave it to the pros. Waxing hurts for a second—and then it's over for two to five weeks. Bonus: The hair that grows back is softer, and there's less of it!

Going the Pro Route

At the waxing salon, you lie down on a table while the operator applies the soft, warm wax with a wooden spatula. She then presses cotton gauze over the wax and, a few seconds later, pulls the cotton up, taking the wax and hair with it. If you do want to splurge and go to a salon, be prepared to pay quite a bit. Prices vary from salon to salon, so it's best to call around.

PHAT Fact

Caffeine makes your skin sensitive, and so does having your period. Can the cola and junk the java for a few hours before you wax and yank.

Other Anti-Hair Methods

Other, more expensive choices for hair removal include …

- ✧ Electrolysis, where a professional "zaps" each hair follicle with an electric current to permanently (or almost permanently) remove the hair. It's painful and expensive.

- ✧ Laser hair removal, which uses a laser to damage the hair follicles to inhibit hair growth. This is not permanent, but it is long term. It's not as painful as electrolysis, but it's extremely expensive—at least a thousand dollars. Unless you've got money to burn and nowhere more meaningful to throw it, stick with some of the other choices.

They say that beauty is only skin deep. We know that's bogus (it's what's underneath that radiates your real beauty), but it's also true that healthy, gorgeous skin looks great and feels great. You may not have a lot of choice in how your skin looks now (those hormones are powerful substances), but even a little skin care now pays off. If not now, later.

The Least You Need to Know

✧ Hormones and heredity make you break out—not what you eat.

✧ Careful cleansing is your first line of defense.

✧ Protect your skin and be aware of any changes.

✧ When it comes to hair removal, know your options!

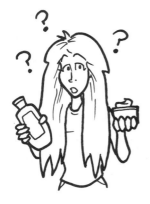

Chapter 15

Looking Great—Hair and Grooming

In This Chapter

✧ Hair for all ethnicities: washing, cutting, and dying

✧ Terrific tips for total tooth care

✧ Man! That's a manicure!

✧ Beating the B.O. baboon

The hair, the teeth, the nails, and the smells!, that's what this chapter is about. You have a lot of grooming choices, and it helps to know the basics—and more. We'll start with the top of the head and move down, down, down.

Hair Here, Hair There

There are almost as many kinds of hair as there are people: flat, full, nappy, curly, bone-straight, wavy, thin, thinning, long and silky, short and spiky, dreadlocked, shaved, purple (or any other groovy color), and many more. And, of course, there's no "right" hair, only hair you feel comfortable with and fantastic flaunting. Here's your head start: Any type of hair looks good if it's healthy and well cared for.

Washing the Locks

No matter what kind of hair you have, it's gonna look crummy when it's filthy. When it comes to hair, clean is good. How often should you wash it? That depends on your own hair.

✧ Wash dry hair no more than once a week with a moisturizing shampoo.

✧ Wash oily hair every day with an oil-absorbing shampoo.

✧ Wash "normal" hair when it needs it—more than once a week and less than every day.

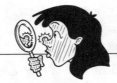

Beautiful? NOT!

Beware the curse of the blow–dryer! Don't cook those curls! Hold the nozzle six inches from your hair and use the low setting. It might take a little longer, but you'll keep your hair shiny and healthy.

Healthy Hair

You have about 100,000 hairs on your head. Each one grows about $1/4$ inch a month. That's why it takes so long for your hair to get long—and if your hair is curly, it seems even longer (all those strands going around and around and around …). You can't stretch your hair, but you can make it healthier and longer-looking … here's how!

✧ Keep it trimmed. Split ends make your hair look shorter, so keep those edges neat.

✧ If you're having grease problems, your hair follicles can plug up, restricting hair growth. You might need to wash your hair more often (like every day).

✧ Keep the blood flowing. As you shampoo, massage your scalp with your fingertips to improve scalp circulation.

✧ Feed your head. If you don't get enough vitamin B_{12} in your diet, your hair's growth can be stunted.

PHAT Fact

Fish, shrimp, spinach, and yogurt all are good sources of vitamin B_{12}, an important nutrient for strong, long hair.

Chopping the Locks

Guys—you usually have it pretty easy. You can always go to a barber (although find one who has a bit of a clue about what's hot and what's not). Girls—hair can be expensive. Hair styling prices start at cheap and go up to ridiculous. What you spend is up to you—and how much you (or your family) are willing to fork out. Remember that expensive doesn't always equal terrific!

Working with a Stylist

Whatever you've got or don't got, when it comes to hair, your stylist can usually make an improvement—if the communication is good! Beware the stylist who tells *you* what *you* want done. How can you find a good stylist? Ask around. Don't be afraid to peer in salon windows and watch the door to see who comes out and how dishy they look.

The Getting-to-Know-You Moment

You've made the appointment or walked in. Now you're sitting in the chair and the stylist starts messing with your hair, getting a feel for the texture and how it falls.

Then he or she starts asking you questions. A good stylist will ask you at least some of the following:

✧ When did you last have your hair cut? And how short was it then?

✧ How often do you change your style?

✧ How much time do you spend on your hair every morning?

✧ Do you do any sports or other activities? Do you have a job after school?

✧ Do you enjoy messing with your own hair?

✧ Do you want your hair style to help disguise any features, like big ears, or a high or low brow line?

✧ And then the million-dollar question: "What would you like me to do today?"

That's the part where I usually sigh and shrug. But you don't have to! Spend a little time before you go (last resort: while you're waiting for your appointment) looking through magazines at hairstyles. Unfortunately, it's not enough to simply decide on a gorgeous hairstyle based on what you see in some fashion mag. The cut's gotta fit the hair—and the face.

Choosing the Look

A good stylist will *know* if the cut you've got your heart set on will work for you. Here are some suggestions for tried-and-true beauty:

✧ For straight, baby-fine hair: Add layers to boost volume, body, and movement (think Christina Aguilera).

✧ For very curly hair: Keep it all one length. Subtle layers at the bottom keep that poofiness to a minimum.

✧ For straight, heavy hair (Asian hair): Regular trims keep long hair sleek and gorgeous. Cut it very short, and you're gonna get that spiky look, even when that's not your intention!

Ethnic Hair, Dyes, and Specialty 'Dos

The world of hair styling is huge, and I can't cover it all. Here are a few special tips and suggestions for making your mane glorious and gorgeous.

African-American Hair

African-American women statistically spend more time, effort, and money on hair than European-American women. Flexible and versatile, African-American hair varies from fine to course, from straight to wavy to very tight, from blond to red to black. African-Americans have a wide variety of styles to choose from: sculptured styles, braids, afros, cornrows, chin length, dreads, and so on.

PHAT Fact

Try a head of mayonnaise for cheap, deep conditioning. Wet your hair slightly, slather the mayo, cover with a plastic shower cap, and heat dry for 15 minutes. Shampoo at least twice to get that greasy slime out.

Did you know that 70 to 90 percent of African-American women use chemical relaxers to straighten, smooth, and soften their hair? Relaxing hair increases its flexibility but also weakens it and tends to dry it out. Watch out for damage and breakage. Keep in mind that African-American hair is sensitive and ...

- ✧ Try not to wash your hair more than once a week or every 10 days to avoid drying it out.
- ✧ Comb and brush gently.

✧ Fluff hair only when damp and easier to comb.

✧ Condition, condition, condition! Using a moisturizing shampoo and heavy conditioners can keep your hair beautiful and healthy.

Asian Hair

About 90 percent of Asians have thick, straight, shiny black or brown hair. It's strong! That strength and beauty also mean that it's reluctant to take a perm or a die job. Asian hair needs very little conditioning. When styling, avoid gels that superhold the hair as these products make Asian hair look stiff (unless you're going for that look). Try leave-in conditioners instead.

Blow-drying can give more control to Asian hair. If it's short, use your fingers to scrunch while drying for more body. If longer, turn the ends under by drying while using a thick, round brush.

Latin Hair

Stylists love to work with Latin hair because it tends to have the strength and glossiness of Asian hair, but most of the time, it's also got some curl or wave to it. It looks great, but it's resistant to straightening or coloring. Unless you want to go red, don't go anywhere. Blow-drying can give more control to Latin hair, too (see the tips in the previous "Asian Hair" section).

Hair Dye Do's and Don'ts

Ask around and you'll hear lots of horror stories about the time Tanya bleached her hair and it all fell out, or Marissa was going for brown and she got green (and not an attractive green, at that!). Serious hair dying is not a do-it-yourself thing (go to a stylist), but there's nothing wrong with playing with temporary (or even semi-permanent) colors—if you do it according to directions. The problem with the less "serious" colors is that they have less effect on those of us with very dark hair. If you're hair dye shopping in a store, *do not* choose the color by the model on the box cover. Look at the back of the box the dye comes in. Sometimes there's a chart that will give you a good indication.

Once your hair has been color-treated, it requires special care to keep the strands healthy. Change your shampoo to one made for color-treated hair.

You can have fun and change your whole look with spray-on hair color in lovely red henna, or, if it will show up without bleaching, brightly colored vegetable dye. Come on, you've always wanted to be a purple head, haven't you? The advantage of these dyes is that they go on easily, they go away when you want them to, and they are gentle on your hair and scalp.

Bad Hair?

Sometimes it seems like there's little worse than a bad hair day. And a bad haircut, permanent, or dye job? Yes, it can bum you out. But be philosophical. Life is not over. You're lucky—it's just hair, and hair grows. Wear a scarf, wear barrettes, wear a wig, wear a hat, or wear your lousy hair with pride. After all, you still have that attitude. You look gorgeous! Before you give up and start wrapping your head like the mummy's long-lost daughter, here are a couple of tips for working with "bad" hair:

- ✧ Make wild, curly hair even wilder. Dampen it, add some conditioner, scrunch it up, and let it fly!

- ✧ If your hair is relatively long, go for the slicked-back pony-tail look. A little gel or pomade goes a long way. It might be a whole new you!

I'm Telling the Tooth!

What about those choppers? There's little more disgusting than a hunk of green or brown wedged into some cutie's teeth or the stained yellow look of a smoker's not-so-pearly whites. The reek of a poorly cleaned mouth is a turn-off for everyone, no matter how hot the rest of the package. To top it off, dental work, while a lot more comfortable than it was in the olden days, is no fun (take it from one who knows), so it's far better to practice a little preventive medicine.

Here's a nightmare image for you: If you leave food on your teeth, germs will gather—millions and millions of them. Together, they form plaque, which creates acid, which eats into the tooth enamel. If you don't brush the plaque away, the tooth begins to decay … and once the decay reaches the inner pulp cavity, the tooth begins to ache and throb.

So, brush!

Brushing your teeth on a regular basis is important for more than the teeth's health—you gotta be thinking about those gums. Gums need care, too, and brushing is a good way to stimulate gum circulation.

PHAT Fact

The main cause of bad breath is bacteria hiding in the pores of your tongue. You can get your tongue professionally scraped; you can buy a tongue scraper; or, you can simply brush your tongue daily with toothpaste and toothbrush.

The Colors of Your Smile

Teeth naturally come in a variety of colors, from pearly blue white to darker ivory. But one thing that's not attractive is tooth stains! Teeth can discolor from coffee or tea, but the worst culprit is nicotine. Those yellow smoking stains are just ugly.

What can you do about it? Whitening toothpastes aren't bleaches, so they can't change the basic color of your teeth. They can help lighten some of the staining. More expensive (and more effective) options include at-home bleaching, a professional solution that costs big bucks, and laser bleaching, done in the dentist's office, which costs even bigger bucks. Best solution? Avoid staining those choppers to begin with.

Nailing It

For some people, polished nails are essential to the "look" they're going for. For others, fingernails just get in the way. You certainly don't *have* to color your nails, but if you're gonna keep them natural, keep them clean and clipped.

When nails get too long and uneven, they get in the way of essential things (like keyboarding and picking up spare change) and they can snag and break and scratch. Even if you want a completely natural look, you might consider using a coat of clear polish to strengthen your nails (and, if you're a nail-biter, to help keep yourself from nibbling).

Giving Yourself a Manicure

A lot of people find giving themselves the occasional manicure to be relaxing, almost like meditating. Plus, you get the bonus of lovely, sleek nails when you're done. Close the door behind you, put on your favorite CD, grab your tools, and settle in! (This can also be a great activity with a friend—you shape together, you soak together, you paint her nails, she paints yours.)

Before you begin: Clean 'em. If your nails have old, peeling polish on them, remove it gently using fingernail-polish remover and cotton balls.

❖ **Step 1: Shape 'em!** Using a fine emery board, file your nails in the shape you choose (oval or squared). Always file in one direction only. Sawing up and down weakens the nail. And never use a metal file—metal causes splitting and peeling.

✧ **Step 2: Soften up!** Apply cuticle cream or lotion to each nail and let it sink in for a couple of minutes.

✧ **Step 3: Soak 'em!** Fill a small bowl with warm water and soak both hands for at least five minutes.

✧ **Step 4: Dry and push.** Dry your hands on the towel; then, using an orange stick, gently push back the cuticles. You can clip a little excess dead skin, but don't cut the cuticles! They guard against infection. My mother used to push her cuticles back with her fingers—gently—every time she washed her hands. She has the most beautiful half-moons around her nails. You can do it with moisturizer or hand cream.

✧ **Step 5: Coat 'em!** Apply moisturizer, rub in, and let dry.

✧ **Step 6: Prep 'em!** Using a base coat, stroke three stripes of polish on each nail (start in the middle of the nail, then add a stroke on either side). It takes some practice to do the "other" hand, so go slow! Make sure your nails have dried before moving on to Step 7.

✧ **Step 7: Polish 'em.** Glide on a coat of your chosen nail color, then wait until it dries completely.

✧ **Step 8: Polish 'em again.**

✧ **Step 9: A clear top coat will seal the job in.** Remember to let them dry completely before using those hands!

✧ **Step 10: Enjoy your glamorous talons!**

The Nail-Biting Blues

A lot of people (including me!) bite their nails. I go through periods of my life when I don't and I have the most gorgeously manicured hands, but most of the time I bite my nails. If you want to stop biting, I know of only three things that will help:

1. **Polish your stubs.** It's unpleasant to bite polished nails, plus, the feel of them makes you stop and think. If you pay for a manicure, you're less likely to bite anyway.

2. **Put evil-tasting stuff on them.** It's available in the drugstore, and it makes your lips pucker from the bitterness. You won't want those fingers in your mouth.

3. **Really want to quit.** If you're ambivalent (feeling two or more ways about it), you won't do it.

Smooth Your Soles

If your feet are feeling rough and neglected, soak them in warm water once a week (the bath is fine), gently rub the calluses on the soles with a pumice stone, exfoliate the rest with a gentle scrub, and then massage them with lotion. Caution: Never use a razor to scrape your feet! They can easily get infected!

Dealing with B.O.

A big part of grooming is smelling good. Nobody likes to talk about it, but sometimes we all stink. B.O. happens because androgen hormones stimulate sweat and oil glands all over your body, particularly in your armpits, hands, feet, back, and crotch. Then, when bacteria grows in these moist, sweaty areas, body odor grows, too! During the teen years when hormones are going bonkers and sweat glands are working hard 24/7, people tend to stink even more. (For girls, hormone levels are highest right before your period begins every month, causing more sweat.)

Smelling-Good Tips

Here are a few tips to keep you smelling sweet:

✧ Keeping clean helps a lot! Wash away that bacteria and odor. Be careful, though, of using antibacterial soap. Some experts believe you need to keep a balance of bacteria—by killing all the bacteria that naturally live in these areas, you invite smellier, hardier ones to move in.

✧ Avoid wearing synthetic materials against your body, particularly in your underwear. Synthetics seal heat and moisture in. Choose cotton, linen, wool, or silk. They do a better job ventilating and absorbing moisture.

✧ Change your socks!

✧ Wash your exercise gear!

✧ Wear a daily deodorant or antiperspirant. What's the difference between them? Deodorants cover up the smell but don't stop the sweating. Antiperspirants seal the skin area (with the chemical aluminum chlor-hydrate) and actually prevent you from perspiring. Some people are sensitive to antiperspirants. If you get a rash, switch to a deodorant!

The Least You Need to Know

✧ Any type of hair looks good if it's healthy and well cared for.

✧ Beware the stylist who tells *you* what *you* want done.

✧ The cut's gotta fit the hair—and the face.

✧ A manicure can be a great way to meditate or hang with a friend.

✧ Beat your B.O. by washing and by wearing natural fibers next to your body.

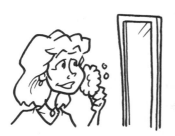

Chapter 16

Working on Your Image, Style, and Makeup

In This Chapter

✦ Looking at image and style

✦ Figuring out your style

✦ Loving—and enhancing—your looks

✦ Shopping—love it or hate it

✦ Putting on your face—makeup tips

In this chapter on style, we'll check out the idea of image, take a look at those people who look good striding down the street in a paper bag, focus on loving your most prominent feature, and get a small handle on shopping. Then it's on to makeup—tips and facts about using it. Yes, this chapter is about stylin', and stylin' is about looking great.

What's Your Image? Where's Your Style?

Whether you're street or jock or granola or stoner or punk or anything in between, you probably have a sense of your own image, how you appear in the world. For teens, how you look and what you wear usually is a statement about what kind of people you hang out with, the music you like, and sometimes, what you like to do.

Bummer! Image Usually Means Judgment

Image is a quick way to tell something about a person, but, unfortunately, it also separates people.

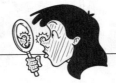

Beautiful? NOT!

Be careful about judging a person by their image. What a person likes is not the same as what a person is like.

When You're Judged

Of course you should be able to wear what you want. But if you're being called a slut because you wear midriff shirts and low-slung shorts, it doesn't feel good. If people think you're a total uptight prude because of what you wear, that doesn't feel good, either. If people stereotype you as a dumb jock because you love sweats, that's pretty awful as well. You're not a slut or a prude or a jock, you're *you*. So how can you use style and fashion to express yourself and really be seen? Part of it might be by wearing different looks.

Image Is Not the Same as Style

Certain people know how to wear anything, and they look great doing it. It's how they walk—that nonchalant, graceful stride. It's the way he wears a cap, she ties a bandana, he knows how to button his shirt so it looks sexy, or how her bangles jangle when she pushes back her hair. If it's not just about what clothes you wear but how you wear them, the million-dollar question becomes, "Can style be learned?" What's style really about?

- ❖ No matter what image you're trying to project, you can look good—and stylish—doing it.
- ❖ Style is about looking the best you can.
- ❖ Style is about asserting your individuality, but also about asserting your membership in a group.
- ❖ Style demonstrates your interests in music, sports, art, and whatever else you do.
- ❖ Style shows your personal tastes in clothing cut, fabric, color, and so on.
- ❖ The same shirt worn by two different people—even people of the same size—can look completely different.
- ❖ At least 80 percent of style is attitude. Confidence looks great.
- ❖ Style can be—but doesn't have to be—expensive.
- ❖ The more chances you take, the more you'll discover your own sense of style.

Finding Style (Where's It Been Hiding?)

Look around you. Take a real look. Take a day and just look at clothing. Here are some questions to start you thinking about your own image and style. Choose a blank page in your "Looking Great" Journal and start writing! There's no right answer. They really are just to make you think. Remember, style and image are attitude-driven.

The Cool and Stylish Quiz

1. What image would you project, and what group would people put you in, if they saw you dressed today?

2. Would this perception change if they saw you yesterday? If so, how?

3. Who's the coolest in your school? What does he or she wear that looks so great?

4. What look can't you stand and why?

5. Write down three things you think about people who wear leather. Would you, could you, should you wear leather?

6. Write down three things you think about people who wear lace. Would you, could you, should you wear lace?

7. Name a garment or look you like but don't think you can wear. Why not?

8. What's your favorite item of clothing? Why?

9. Choose one: comfort or beauty. Why?

Boosting Your Style, Boosting Your Beauty

There are three billion types of beauty, and true sexiness comes from the inside out. It's all about attitude and style. One trick to finding your style—and looking beautiful with it—is finding your favorite feature and focusing in on it.

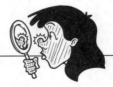

Beautiful? NOT!

Don't get sucked in! Fashion magazines can help you determine what kind of "look" you're going for. Remember, though, that magazines give an unrealistic view of what women and girls look like.

Your "Looking Great" Features Exercise

For every feature on your face (eyes, nose, cheeks, lips, chin, forehead, brows, and so on), write something positive. Start with its function, "My nose smells," and move on from there. Focusing on the positive is actually powerful medicine —the human brain is an amazing feature (ooh ... did you include your brain in the exercise?). If you tell it something long enough, it begins to believe it.

Boosting Your Features

Finding what's special about your looks and stressing them is key to looking great. Here are some ideas for you, especially if you have some features that aren't always considered gorgeous (hey, don't we all?):

- ✦ **Love your pale, pale skin?** Isn't it creamy and smooth, glowing from within? Go for a foundation that matches your skin tone exactly (or go completely without, you lucky dawg).

- ✦ **Braces are beautiful!** (Yes, really!) Stop hiding them behind those closed lips. With those braces, you're *sooo* cute!

- ✦ **Wear those wide-set eyes with pride.** Wide-set eyes are the look of 1940s movie-screen queens and look great with side parts. Go for earth tones in your eye makeup.

- ✦ **Thick, thicker, thickest brows.** Shape them, yes, but don't pluck or wax them off! If you want to play with them, just shape them up a bit, and get rid of the stray hair. Brush them upward and out with a toothbrush (yes, you can use a brow gel, but an eeny touch of petroleum jelly will do as well).

- ✦ **Great glasses.** Glasses magnify your eyes, and your eyes are the windows to your soul. Glasses are the ultimate accessory, say the style setters. They're an invisible barrier that teases and delights (look at what Nicole Kidman wore to the Oscars).

219

✧ **Freakin' fantastic freckles** ... Charming, sexy, delight-
ful, one of a kind ... Nobody's freckles are like yours.
Don't cover them up with foundation and concealer. If
you use a foundation, make sure it's translucent so that
you're simply evening up the skin tone without covering your little dots.

✧ **Big-nose beauty?** So, your nose is big? A big nose is a
sign of beauty, character, sexiness, and nobility (think
Sarah Jessica Parker). Pamper its glory—don't minimize
it. Noses collect oil and blackheads, so make sure to
clean well (see Chapter 14, "The Skin You're In").

✧ **Big juicy lips?** Well aren't you lucky?! People pay good
money for those. Keep them plump and healthy.

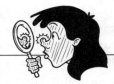

Beautiful? NOT!

Goop, gunk, and leftovers do not look great in braces.
Make sure you brush after every meal, carry a toothpick
for emergencies, and master the furtive mirror-check move
to verify that your spinach hasn't taken up permanent resi-
dence.

Get Dressed!

The most fashionable, cool, hip, sophisticated people in the
world are not the most beautiful. But what these people do
have is style, and a sense of what looks good on them.

What Looks Good? What Do You Like?

They used to say that heavy people should never wear hori-
zontal stripes, that tall, skinny people should break up their

long lines with belts and color, and that black was the finest thing for slimming. If you've got a fairly average-size and -shape body (shut up! So what if you think your thighs are a size too big and your bust a size too small!), you don't need to apply these kinds of rules. Leather, lace, prints, solids, stripes—it's up to you to decide. Remember that it's not just what looks "good" on you, it's what you *like*. Try it on. Ask yourself:

◈ Does it fit? Does it pull, pinch, bag, sag, stretch, strain, or hang like a sack? I promise you—if it doesn't hang right, it doesn't have style.

◈ Does it feel good on you? Do you like touching the fabric?

◈ Is it comfortable? If it's not, you're gonna be pretty grumpy.

◈ Do you feel attractive in it? Do you feel very attractive? Do you feel too attractive? (Too attractive can be scary.)

◈ What do other people think? Ask your friends, or ask your mom—*if* you trust her opinion.

◈ No matter what others think, what do you think?

PHAT Fact

Think that outfit is made for that skinny model in the magazine? Chances are, she's too thin. I wish you could see all the safety pins in the back, stretching the dress up against her body.

Chillin' with Colors

Styles in colors change from year to year and from decade to decade (and I recently heard somebody say that the color of the new millennium is blue). Come on! By the time you're in your teens, you probably have a good idea of some of the colors that look good on you—they're the ones you're wearing when people compliment you. You might also have an idea of some of the colors that don't look good on you.

Doing your colors became a fad a while ago, and if you go into any library, you'll be able to find books about how to figure out what "season" you are and what colors look best on you. Once you know your colors (or pay to have your colors done), you can go into any store and start choosing clothes by which ones are in the most flattering colors for you.

He Sez

"I try not to pay too much attention to style, but it is a big factor in people's lives—they want to look good in public. I don't want to go out with my hair all weird or anything, but I think it's more of a girl thing than a guy thing."

—Josh, age 14

Shopping Smart and Shopping Cheap

One thing about teens: They don't always have a lot of money. And even if they do, they like to spread it around. That's why it's so important to shop smart and to shop cheap.

At the Mall

Whether it's Old Navy or The Gap or a smaller boutique, you'll no doubt find the look you're looking for at the mall.

But does shopping at the mall make sense money-wise? It does if you have lots of money or lots of time to wait for sales on the items you want. Most of the stores rarely, if ever, put their old standards on sale—the classic jeans, for instance. It's usually the seasonal clothes—once they're out of season. Which isn't fair for teens, because if you're still growing, you can't wait for a year to wear that summer shirt—it might not fit you. Plus, it might be long out of style.

The good thing about shopping at the mall is that so much of the clothing is geared and designed for teens. That means it's easy to find clothing that looks good and that's stylin'. It's paying for it that's the problem.

PHAT Fact

It's all ads! Almost every tip you find in a magazine is geared to make you buy products. Even if you never had to think about money, nobody has room in the bathroom cabinet for all those lotions and potions.

Consignment, Thrift, and Vintage

Consignment shops and thrift shops are a great option for teens looking for clothes (and to satisfy that urge to shop even when the funds are a little low). Shopping bonuses:

- ✧ You can try on all sorts of different looks (hats, belts, shoes, too!) and develop your own sense of style.

- ✧ You can afford lots more clothes. If you think about the comparison in prices, buying retail is insane!

- ✧ You can get that slightly funky, endlessly hip look almost without trying.

> ✧ If you're like me and get slightly dazed and claustrophobic in big stores, you'll feel less overwhelmed.

> ✧ It's fun, and it's a great activity to do with a friend.

PHAT Fact

It's school shopping time. One expensive item or three cheapies? Your mom's arguing for the expensive item. It's durable, it's a classic. But you're growing, and you stain things. I say go for the cheapies and get three kicky looks.

Makeup Tips for Every Type

You can use makeup to conceal or to reveal or to create an image. You can also use makeup to change an image temporarily. When you're ready for a change in your life, changing your look can be a quick, cheap cure for the blahs.

Healthy Stuff for Your Skin

You can buy a whole lot of junk to put on your skin, but you might be adding to breakouts, clogged pores, or even worse! There's lots more on skin care in Chapter 14, but if you're wearing makeup, make sure you ...

> ✧ Watch out for products containing lanolin (it clogs your pores). If you're breaking out from your makeup, go for allergy-tested or sensitive-skin products. They might be more expensive, but the idea is to look great, right? Zits don't look great.

> ✧ Clean it off! Models spend almost as much time taking their makeup off as they do putting it on.

✧ Clean your tools. Makeup brushes and puffs collect oil and bacteria from your skin. Besides the yuckiness of all that grease and germs, they just won't work as well, and they might muddy up your colors. To clean brushes, soak them in warm water with baby shampoo or liquid dishwashing soap for 10 or 15 minutes. Rinse, towel blot dry, and let sit until dry. If you use makeup every day, you should clean your tools every couple of weeks.

She Sez

"My mom doesn't wear a lot of makeup—she's an architect—but I've noticed that all the secretaries in her office do. Seems like the more power you have as a woman in this society, the less you have to dress and look like a doll."

—Sandy, age 18

Don't Break That Bank, Baby!

The cosmetic industry is huge, and everybody wants a piece of your dollar. It can be a trap! If you're into makeup, inexpensive cosmetics are fine. If you want to blow some cash, spend it on makeup tools: a few good powder puffs (change them every few months), a good triangular sponge or two, and some makeup brushes. The pros spend hundreds of dollars on sable hair brushes. They're nice, but ...

Foundation and Concealer

Foundation, the base of it all, is not usually necessary for teens. If you decide to use it, be careful! Plain and simple,

225

foundation looks horrendous when done wrong. Celebrate your natural skin tones (no matter *how* broken out you are), and let them shine through. Foundation makeup—makeup of all kinds—is to add to your natural beauty, not build a wall to step behind.

The primary "crime" of foundation is applying it too heavily. Yeah, you want to disguise and cover those zits, and double yeah, you want to even out those skin tones. But that's it! And really, that's the purpose of concealers.

Concealers are for spot control—that zit, that blotch, that odd mark. Match your concealer carefully—your best bet is the makeup counter at a department store where the sales-

PHAT Fact

Always apply foundation to clean skin. If your skin is oily or overly dry in spots, the foundation will clump and look blotchy.

person can help you. And be prepared—makeup isn't cheap. A tube of the right color concealer should last you for a good, long time, though.

I've Got My Eye(Shadow) on You!

They say that the eyes are the windows to the soul, and the right touch of subtle eye makeup can enhance and create mystery. Here are a couple of "eye-catching" tips:

✧ Try curling your lashes for a quick, yet dramatic emphasis on your peepers.

✧ Apply your eye shadow with the most at the outside of the eye, the least at the nose.

✧ Before you apply, make sure that your eyelids are clean and oil-free.

✧ Powder eye shadow is easier to handle and won't clump up in the creases.

✧ Pat your lids with a touch of matte foundation to help the shadow glide on smoothly.

✧ For rich, natural impact, use earthy greens and browns instead of pastels.

Give Me Some Lip!

What's the world's most common item of makeup? Lipstick! Wearing lip color alone can give a great look, so long as the color goes with your skin tones. (Lip color without any other makeup tends to over-emphasize the lips and throw the whole face out of balance. Look for a shade of lipstick that flatters your skin, rather than "pops.")

She Sez

"I like my black lipstick and purple toenail polish. It's so different from my normal, more natural look. It's like putting on a costume; I can step outside of myself and get away from it all."

—Rita, age 17

PHAT Fact

Always remove your mascara first, with either a little oil and a cotton swab or a nonoily makeup remover. Water-proof mascara is a pain to take off—so don't use it unless you're going swimming; to a tear-jerker, a wedding, a funeral; or are planning a big breakup.

Style—It's Your Choice

No matter what your wear, how you wear it, where you buy it, or how you apply it, it's all only important as a reflection of who you are inside. Play with style. It's your chance to try on who you want to be.

The Least You Need to Know

✧ What you wear might tell something about what you *like,* but it doesn't tell what you *are like.*

✧ No matter what your image, you can have style. It's attitude and knowing what looks good on you.

✧ Emphasize the parts of you that are unusual.

✧ When you're buying clothes, *try them on!!*

✧ Vintage and used clothing stores are a great solution for teens with style but little cash.

✧ Makeup can help you create an image.

Part 6

Dealing with the Uglies

Hormones and stress: the teenager's nightmare, the teenager's reality. It's hard to look great when you're bummed out, over-worked, under-appreciated, and (if you're a girl), dealing with PMS on top of it all. To look your best, you need some calm and serenity. This section is designed to help you chill out. You'll get specific tools to help you deal with what's bugging you. Read carefully—life will feel blissful again!

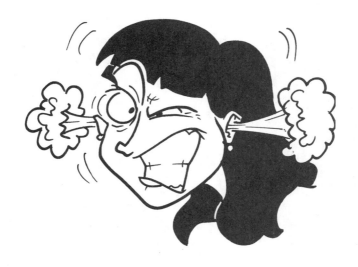

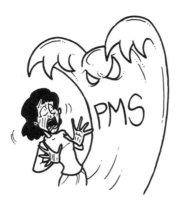

Chapter 17

Attack of the Hormones!

In This Chapter

◇ Looking at the ties between hormones, your period, and food

◇ Calcium and PMS blahs: Could it cure?

◇ Looking—and feeling—great during your period

◇ Protecting yourself from pregnancy and disease

Being a teen is, in large part, about hormones. Hormones affect your waking thoughts, your dreams, your desires, and your relationships. Hormones also affect your sleep patterns, your moods, your skin, your eating habits, and your exercise patterns.

This chapter is mostly about girls' hormonal cycles, including information on eating, exercise and PMS; your period; and birth control. Whoa! If you're a guy, don't leave! It's important to understand how the other gender is put together.

Hormones and FOOD

Hormonal surges make you moody. So does ...

✧ Skipping breakfast.

✧ Eating a lot of sugar or drinking a lot of caffeine—you might feel fine for a while, but later on you will experience a big slump.

✧ Hating yourself because you're overeating or starving yourself.

✧ And so on ...

So, if you think about it, combining the normal moodiness of being a teen with the not-so-great eating behaviors I just mentioned can lead to even more—and more extreme—mood swings. What's the logical conclusion? Chill with the lousy eating, and be kind to your body!

PHAT Fact

Chart your cycles. The average menstrual cycle is 28 days. Your cycle might be longer or shorter, or vary; a lot of teens are irregular. Keeping track of when you get your period is the first step to understanding your rhythms. (I put a dot on the calendar.)

If you have PMS (more on this to follow) or painful periods (more on this later, too), there are a number of remedies that might help you feel better. Try some of the following (and keep in mind that every body is different):

✧ Cut down on salty foods before and during your period. That means chips, pretzels, soy sauce, salted nuts, spicy foods, and so on. The problem with eating a lot of salt (just when you're craving it most) is that it makes you retain water, leading to that bloated, puffy feeling.

✧ Some herbal teas (like raspberry leaf) can help relieve cramps.

✧ For the 10 or so days before your period, watch your sugar intake, and cut down on caffeine, sugar, and white flour. Okay, you're screaming at me, "Hey! That about covers all I eat!" Go back, back, back to the earlier chapters in this book. Also know that you're probably not going to be able to cut back on all of these things completely. (You're human, you know.)

✧ Ban the booze. Alcohol can increase cramping and headaches during your period. For some reason, wine and beer are worse than other alcoholic beverages (no, that *doesn't* mean you should switch to vodka!).

PHAT Fact

Women who get PMS usually do not have severe cramping during their periods. Well, at least that's something positive about it!

The PMS Reduction Recipe

It's known as PMS (premenstrual syndrome) or turning into a complete and raving lunatic. Looking great is a little tricky if you're a raving lunatic.

Do you have PMS?

> ✧ Is it the week before your period?

And ...

> ✧ Are you moody, depressed, and/or agitated?
>
> ✧ Are you bloated?
>
> ✧ Are your breasts tender?
>
> ✧ Are you getting headaches?
>
> ✧ Do you feel irrational?
>
> ✧ Do you cry at the drop of a hat?
>
> ✧ Are you constipated?
>
> ✧ Are you tending to gain weight?
>
> ✧ Do you crave salt, chocolate, or specific foods more than you usually do the rest of the month?

If you have some or all of these symptoms ... welcome! Join the ranks of women and girls who get PMS.

PMS is pretty specific. It's a collection of symptoms that occur in the 10 days between ovulation and getting your period. PMS might be mild or it might be a total terror that hits you once a month. The upside? The minute you get your period, you tend to feel better.

Dealing with It—the Calcium Solution

Ann O'Connor, my wise and wonderful GYN Nurse Practitioner at Kaiser Hospital in Oakland, California, says the best way to eliminate PMS is to make sure you're getting enough calcium. Half of all women and girls who up their calcium intake will see their PMS symptoms come to a total stop (and that's pretty great!). Other solutions include vitamin D, vitamin B_6, and magnesium.

Considering Your Calcium

The average teen is deficient in calcium. You need at least 1,200 milligrams of the stuff, which you can get by drinking a quart of milk a day. Yes, you read right, a QUART. If you feel like that much would choke a horse—let alone you—or if you're lactose intolerant (more on this to follow), consider taking calcium supplements. Here's what to look for:

✧ Tums, Rolaids, Os-Cal and other calcium carbonate products are the least expensive. Check the label to find out how much calcium is included (it's under the name "elemental calcium.")

✧ Also check out Viactiv, a low-fat caramel with lots of calcium (it also has milk, so if you're allergic, avoid this product!). One or two of these a few times a day and yum! ... I mean ... bravo for the calcium!

✧ Products with Calcium Gluconate, Calcium Lactate, and Calcium Citrate have less calcium per tablet than those made with calcium carbonate, so you might need to take more of them to get your recommended daily dosage.

While we're at it, don't forget that cola leaches calcium from the kidneys and caffeine keeps calcium from being absorbed.

PHAT Fact

Your body needs vitamin D to absorb calcium. Milk is fortified with it ... but if you're not getting your calcium from milk, you might need to supplement with tablets or capsules.

It's Not Just in Milk!

Remember back in Chapter 3 when we looked at sources of calcium? Again, here's that list of calcium-rich foods: tofu, spinach, artichokes, rhubarb, beet greens, kale, beans, chick peas, pumpkin, and sweet potatoes. Oops! I forgot the calcium-fortified orange juice! (And if you like them, sardines—with the bones—are pretty terrific, too.)

Lactose, Sit Down! I Cannot Tolerate You!

Some people feel sick when they eat milk products. They get gassy, bloat, get cramps or diarrhea. This is called lactose intolerance. Try …

✧ Eating smaller amounts of milk products at a time.

✧ Cottage cheese or yogurt.

✧ Lactose tolerance products like Lactaid milk (treated to improve your tolerance), Lactaid drops (you add them to your milk), Lactaid tablets (you eat them with milk products) or Dairy Ease (a chewable tablet).

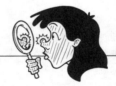

Beautiful? NOT!

Don't forget the vitamin C! Without vitamin C, your body cannot absorb calcium. Drink that OJ or supplement with tablets during the PMS week.

Vital Vitamins and Magnificent Magnesium

Once you've gotten your calcium up, check out how you feel for a couple of months. Still having PMS symptoms? Here are some other things to try:

✧ **Vitamin B$_6$.** 50 milligrams a day (be cool and forget about large doses of this stuff, they can be dangerous!)

✧ **Vitamin E.** 400 IU a day. Vitamin E is great for breast tenderness.

✧ **Magnesium.** It soothes the nerves and that awful jangy clangy kind of energy.

Whoops!!! Cut Yourself Some Slack

"Remember that your coordination can be off during the PMS week," says Ann O'Connor, N.P., "especially when you're trying to do a new skill. You're more uncoordinated. It's more complicated; you drop things. If you have to do driving lessons during that week, especially if you're learning a stick shift, don't be discouraged if they don't go as well."

PMS and Exercise

Especially if you suffer from feeling sluggish and bloated during your PMS week, it can be hard to convince yourself that your body really needs to get out there and exercise. Guess what! It does. It might be hard to get motivated, but once you're out there you'll feel better, and exercise during the PMS week leads to fewer cramps once "Auntie" finally arrives.

Looking/Feeling Great When "Auntie" Comes to Town

Once your PMS week is over, you get your period. Some teen girls, especially girls who suffer from cramps during their period, want nothing more than to crawl into bed with a heating pad and pull the covers over their head. Maybe mom will bring you a cup of hot milk … and where's the acetaminophen? Yes, a hot water bottle can help cramps, but there are other ways to deal with—and even avoid—discomfort.

Your Period and Exercise

Having your period might not affect you during exercise, or it might make you feel bloated, sluggish, or tired. If you're feeling crampy, the last thing you might want to do is get up and work out. Force yourself.

Some women feel weaker during their period. This doesn't mean you should sideline yourself. Exercise during your period can help you avoid getting cramps, reduces cramps if you do get them, and actually can increase your energy. Here are a couple of tips:

⬦ If you're feeling bloated, wear looser clothes (with the exception of the following), and take it a little slower.

⬦ Worried about leaking during your period? If you have heavy periods and are concerned about exercising, consider bike shorts, a pad and a tampon.

She Sez

"My friend Megan is not athletic—not at all. It, like, kills her to exercise. When she has her period, she tells the gym teacher; and *she* says, 'It's good for you to exercise.'"

—Arden, age 13

Your Period and Cramp Relief

Some teens cramp severely, some never get cramps, and some get some cramping sometimes. Cramping tends to get better as you get older. While you're waiting for time to take its course, here are some suggestions to help you feel better:

⬦ Relax your body. Yeah, right! I know, you're all cramped up, so there you are doubled over on the bed, in pain, and tense as can be. Tenseness usually is rooted in fear. Reassure yourself that cramping is a normal part of this menstrual process, and there's nothing wrong with your body.

✧ Use deep breathing to calm your body down.

✧ Curl your body around a hot water bottle or heating pad. The knee-to-chest, fetal position can feel very soothing. Or, lie on your back and hug your knees to your chest.

✧ Hit somebody up for a back rub, and have them focus on your tailbone area.

✧ Gently massage your abdomen while breathing deeply.

✧ For many women, being sexually aroused or having an orgasm can help relieve pain and start the flow of your period (you don't need a partner for this).

✧ Aspirin, Midol, or acetaminophen.

Healthy Sexuality

Teens are intensely sexual beings. It's part of that puberty stuff, and it's part of becoming an adult. Your desires rage, your body aches for love, and your mind seems obsessed. It's important to understand your sexual feelings; your sexuality is part of who you are as a human being. But whatever your sexuality, it's also important to understand that ...

✧ Sexual feelings feel good, but you don't have to act them out with other people.

✧ Most people get into "trouble" with sex because they have poor impulse control—that means they pretty much go to it when their body tells them to.

✧ Your sexuality is your own. It takes time to understand what you like and dislike. Make sex a conscious decision—don't just slide into it.

✧ Sex and sexuality doesn't just mean intercourse. There are many ways to be a sexual person without "doin' it."

✧ It's vital to protect yourself—from pregnancy, disease, negative or pressured situations, or doing things you feel troubled or concerned about.

Preventing Pregnancy and Sexually Transmitted Diseases (STDs)

Birth control prevents pregnancy. There are several basic types of birth control methods, the main ones being the barrier methods (condoms, diaphragms, the sponge), the chemical methods (spermicidal foam, jellies, and cream) and the hormonal methods, like the pill and the depo-provera shot.

Barrier methods include the diaphragm (which helps prevent pregnancy) and the condom (both male and female condom) which help prevent both pregnancy and STDs. Barrier control methods can be very effective in preventing pregnancy if used correctly every single time. Some, like the condom, also help prevent STDs.

PHAT Fact

Here's a scary thought: Without using birth control, four out of five couples having intercourse will get pregnant in the first year! Protect yourself, every time!

What's Best?

Choosing a form of birth control and disease protection is a personal decision. Here are some facts that will help:

✧ Abstinence (no sex with another person) is utterly effective in preventing both pregnancy and STDs.

✧ Nonintercourse lovemaking (oral sex and mutual masturbation) is fairly effective at preventing pregnancy, as long as the penis doesn't get anywhere near the vagina. It's not as effective in preventing STDs, because germs can be transmitted through cuts, sperm, vaginal secretions, and menstrual blood.

✧ A condom used with a spermicide is the best form of birth control for sexually active teens. It's cheap, effective, provides STD protection, and has no side effects.

✧ Hormonal birth control methods can be very effective in preventing pregnancy, but if you use one of them, you have to understand that they strongly affect your hormonal levels, and your hormones affect your mood, your weight, your skin … your everything. They also need to be used with a condom to prevent STDs.

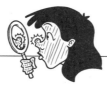

Beautiful? NOT!

The pill, the shot, the IUD, the diaphragm, the cap … what do they have in common? They all help prevent pregnancy, but they *don't* protect against STDs (sexually transmitted diseases) including AIDS. You need a barrier method to protect against STDs. The best prevention? Condoms.

Name That STD!

Alas, there are a lot of sexually transmitted diseases (STDs). Some are more dangerous than others—AIDS kills people—but all require medical attention. You can catch STDs from friends and strangers. Having—and transmitting—STDs isn't limited to people who sleep around, look dog-like, or have reputations. Anyone who is sexually active can have an STD.

For more information on STDs, call the STD Hotline at the Centers for Disease Control. They have a toll-free number: 1-800-227-8922.

And here's a list of some of the diseases you can get from unsafe sex: Gonorrhea, Syphilis, Chlamydia, HIV/AIDS, Hepatitis A, B, and C, Herpes, HPV (Genital Warts), Vaginal Infections, Parasites (Pubic Lice or Crabs). Protect yourself! Every time!

The Least You Need to Know

✧ Your moods and hormones are linked, and both are linked to what you eat.

✧ Getting enough calcium cures PMS in 50 percent of women who try it.

✧ Exercise really helps to relieve both PMS and period symptoms.

✧ The hormonal birth control methods do more than just keep you from getting pregnant. They also affect your moods, looks, and how you feel physically.

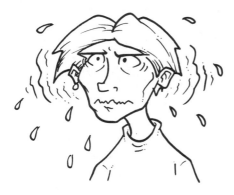

Chapter 18

Stress Busting

In This Chapter

✧ So ... why are *you* so stressed out?

✧ The move-your-body solution

✧ Why you're so tired, and why that's not so bad

✧ Tips and tricks for stress reduction

✧ Dealing with depression

✧ The meaning of life

> **Q:** Why is there a chapter on handling stress in a health and beauty book?
>
> **A:** Because stress directly impacts your health, your eating, your sleeping, your hormones, your skin, your posture ... in short, all the things that make you look great ... or not.

This chapter is about taking care of yourself, pampering yourself, nurturing yourself. When you reduce the stress in your life—when you feel better—you tend to look better, too.

What Happens When You're Stressed?

Stress doesn't just happen in your brain, it happens in your body, too. Your body holds stress in your muscles (that's why your neck is so tight!). It makes it hard to sleep, and to even deal with life. You might get angry, irritable, or depressed—or all of these. You might get indigestion. Everybody gets stressed out by different things, and everybody reacts to stress in their own way.

Mood Swings, Hormones, Family and School Pressures

Being a teen is tough. School is demanding; you're working and doing extracurricular stuff in the cracks, and your schedule is very tight. Puberty brings mood swings and hormonal surges, and it often brings real changes in your family's dynamics. No wonder you're not always serene!

She Sez

"I have a lot of stress in my life. I get home from school, run to soccer practice, do homework, have dinner, practice piano. Calling up a friend helps. Writing helps—what I've done, what's getting on my nerves, what guys I like."

—Arden, age 13

What's Winding Your Chain?

Here are some of the stresses teens commonly face:

✧ The big time crunch. You simply don't have enough time.

- ✧ The social crunch. Trying to be yourself and fit in. Trying to avoid being categorized as a punk, prep, goth, nerd, druggie, jock, skater, brain, alternative, geek, loser, slut, stud, freak, poser …

- ✧ Your parents. The struggle to get them to see you as you.

- ✧ School pressure. You have so much riding on these years. And what happens if you mess up?

- ✧ Your love life, or lack of it.

- ✧ External pressures. Sexual harassment, money worries, racial profiling … the sad, sad state of the world can easily get you down.

- ✧ Your looks. Your skin, weight, development, hair, build, style …

- ✧ … and so on, and so on, and so on.

PHAT Fact

You might not know what you're feeling, except confused! Emotions don't always wait in line, neatly, and take turns. Sometimes it's a mosh pit: anger, happiness, boredom, love, fear, anxiety, pride, jealousy, grief, horniness, loneliness … all crowding in, screaming for attention.

Get It off Your Chest!

… or call a buddy, or write a long, intense e-mail. Chat rooms can be good for venting steam, too (especially because you can be anonymous if you like). It's important to express your feelings, whether it's to a friend, your "Looking Great" Journal, or a stranger on the Web.

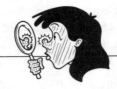

Beautiful? NOT!

Be careful to avoid giving out your personal information to people you meet online. You've heard the horror stories—they're true! People aren't always what they seem. Play it safe.

Exercise Helps!

Running it off, the comradery of a hard basketball game, pumping iron alone in your room, performing in a school dance show, all of these—any form of exercise—can dramatically lower your stress and depression levels.

The Bio-Medical Explanation

Exercise actually makes you feel good. That's not just because you get a sense of accomplishment from moving your body and getting in shape. No ... blame it on the endorphins, a brain chemical released when you exercise. Exercise actually works to improve your mood!

But Not Obsessive Exercise

But that doesn't mean too much exercise. Exercise can become an addiction, just like drugs (I guess you get hooked on that endorphin rush). Exercise can be a distraction from daily life. A little distraction is fine—it's great, actually—but exercising to an extreme can injure your body and serve as a way to avoid life.

Sleep! Special Teen Rhythms and Issues

When you were a kid, you got up when your parents told you to; you had a standard bedtime (although you probably tried to stay up past it). Now, everybody's on your back because you like to sleep, and you like to sleep until noon. They're calling you lazy. You're tired in the morning—but then you come alive at night, just when everybody else is settling in. What's up with that?

Teenagers have different sleep needs. As in, you need a lot! You're not lazy, you're growing. When you don't sleep enough, all sorts of horrific problems can occur:

✧ Your skin looks lousy

✧ It's hard to concentrate, impossible to focus

✧ You become forgetful

✧ You show poor judgment ("I can fly off that tall building!")

✧ You get clumsy and klutzy

✧ You get moody, broody, and overly emotional

Give yourself permission to hours of sleep! No, you can't get by on a regular schedule of six hours sleep a night and catching up on the weekend. That kind of catching up doesn't work. You never do catch up; plus, if you oversleep one day, you'll find it harder to sleep the next day.

PHAT Fact

When you don't get enough sleep, you get stressed out and exhausted. When you're stressed out, it's hard to sleep. How's that for an evil cycle?

It's best to schedule your life so you can sleep, and keep your sleep patterns as rhythmic as possible.

Soothing Out the Stress

Stressed out and feeling lousy? It's time to treat yourself right. Learning to do soothing things for yourself can help you get through life's hard times.

"I Vant to Be Alone!"

Some people like to be alone, and some people don't.

For introverts, a walk in nature, a quiet afternoon in your bedroom with a book, or a long, quiet bath can help de-stress your body and mind. For extroverts, an afternoon hanging with your friends can do the same thing.

She Sez

"When I'm by myself, it doesn't help me. I just get more mad and sad when I'm alone. Really it's just me cutting myself off. I just feel more mad that I'm left out. It's better that I go talk to somebody else."

—Arden, age 13

Yoga-riffic

The East Indian practice of yoga, a series of alignment and stretching exercises (with a life philosophy behind it) helps you relax and focus, as well as stretch out your muscles. It's an excellent stress reducer. Check out local yoga classes— they range from very easy and slow to high-powered and demanding.

Breathe! Force Yerself to Relax, Baby!

When you're wound up tight, it's seductive to stay that tight. You might be scared that if you let yourself relax, everything will fall apart. It won't. When you relax, when you reduce the stress in your body, you're a lot better equipped to handle the things that are getting you so tight. And one way to relax your body is to practice deep breathing.

You can breathe deeply anywhere. When you focus on your breath, you empty your mind (similar to meditation). You also bring more oxygen into your body. It's energizing and relaxing.

Breathe in deeply through your nose. Let the breath flow all the way down to your tummy (not just into your chest). Release the breath through your mouth. Repeat. Don't hold your breath—you might get light-headed.

Meaningful Meditation

Meditation reduces high blood pressure and lowers stress—it's a medically proven fact. Meditation simply means sitting quietly and emptying your mind of thoughts for a while.

Get yourself comfortable while sitting on the floor, your back straight, your legs crossed. Close your eyes. Quiet your mind. Let the thoughts breeze in and out as you breathe through your nose. Focus on your breathing. Don't think about the time. Focus on now, on the moment, on your breathing. If your thoughts wander, don't go with them … stay focused on the moment.

Some people use a simple word or phrase as something to concentrate on while meditating.

The Self-Spa Treatment

Doing nice things for yourself and your body can help reduce your stress. Here are a couple of ways to pamper yourself.

A Tropical Home Facial

Feeling like a bit of the tropics? (Balmy winds ... gentle waves ... warm sand ...)

Try this recipe:

> 1 banana (overripe is fine)
>
> $1/2$ avocado (save the rest for a delicious snack with a squeeze of lemon)
>
> 2 tablespoons honey

Wash your face well. Combine the ingredients in a bowl. Mash well until they're all incorporated together. Sit in a comfortable position with your hair tied back if it's long, and a towel around your neck. Smooth the mixture on your clean face. Don't lick your lips! After 20 minutes, rinse it off. Now go enjoy your snack.

The Incredible, Edible Citrus Bath

With a bag of fruit and some warm water, you can transform your bathroom into a tropical palace.

Recipe:

> 3 lemons
>
> 3 oranges
>
> 1 bathtub

Cut three lemons and three oranges in half. Fill your bathtub with warm water and squeeze the fruit into the bathtub. Now slice the fruit and toss it in. Settle in, sink down, relax, and soak for 20 minutes. Remember to rinse! Note: don't try this if drinking orange juice gives you a rash!

When You're Feeling Soooo Blue ...

Being a teen has a dark side. Sometimes it's not just moods. Sometimes you really are depressed, abusing drugs, yourself or somebody else, acting out sexually or with bad behavior, or suffering from an eating disorder. You might be turning in on yourself and self-injuring.

Self-Injury

When you take all that stress and depression and suck it down, it sometimes comes out through self-injury.

PHAT Fact

There are a hecka lot of people in the United States who self-injure. Wanna try around two million? That's what the experts say!

Self-injury means cutting yourself, burning yourself, and/or extreme risk-taking as an attempt to relieve extreme anxiety. Because many self-injurers hide their deeds (sliced arms under long sleeves, cigarette burns on your chest or bottom), you might think you're the only one who's ever invented such a terrible behavior. The first thing to know is, you're not the only one ... no, you're not weird! Unfortunately, self-injury is an extremely common—though not a very effective or self-loving—way to handle stress. And yes, you can get some help to stop; check out the resources in the appendix.

Down, Dirty, and Depressed

You feel low. You feel hopeless, tired, sleepless, and anxious. This might not be the ordinary teen blahs and moodiness ... you might be depressed. According to the Center for Mental Health Services (they're part of the U.S. Department of Health and Human Services), close to 13 percent of all teen-agers are clinically depressed.

You might be depressed because of something in your life, or you might just be depressed without having a specific reason.

What makes it worse is the fact that people usually don't think of teens as depressed. Some adults have the bogus idea that the high school years are the best years of your life (believe me, they're not!). Adults tend to diminish teen love problems (puppy love!) and stress overload ("Wait until you have to *work* for a living!"). They don't understand that it's a hard time in life. And they often don't believe that teens can even get depressed.

Symptoms of Depression

Here are some of the symptoms you might have if you're depressed. Keep in mind that each of these things could be caused by something else: irritability, rage, moodiness, disruptive or violent behavior (toward others or yourself), unexplained fears, a preoccupation with death, trouble sleeping, a change in your interests or a loss of interests.

Are you getting a lot of stomach aches or headaches? Are you tired all the time? (Are there other reasons for these symptoms?)

Are you "self-medicating" with drugs or alcohol to make yourself feel better? (Depressed teens are at a higher risk for drug or alcohol abuse.)

PHAT Fact

Depression is a medical diagnosis. You can't diagnose your own depression! If you have a lot of depressed symptoms, don't assume you are truly clinically depressed. You should definitely check it out with your doctor.

Fix Me, Doc!

Depression is treatable! Facing your depression helps. Talking about it helps. Writing about it helps. Learning to cope with it helps. Realizing you'll live through it helps.

If you are diagnosed as depressed, you'll be treated with psychotherapy, drug therapy, or both. The main idea is to help you feel better, to solve your problems, and to get "unstuck."

Psychotherapy is "talk" therapy. You'll see a therapist or psychiatrist, and work with him or her to talk out what's bugging you in your life and find solutions to your problems. Nobody will ever force you to say anything, and nobody will force you to do anything. What you say to a therapist remains completely confidential (that means they can't tell anybody—including your parents!). Actually, that's not quite true—if they feel you're in danger of hurting yourself or somebody else, then they'll let the "authorities" know. But your inner secrets are safe. It's the law.

When you're on drug therapy, you'll probably be seeing a therapist for talk therapy, too. You might be given medications to help you sleep and calm your anxiety. These change your mood—they don't change your personality. Most teens don't need drug therapy, although it can be very, very effective in helping you feel better.

Finding a Purpose

This book has focused on you, but so much of feeling good about yourself ultimately depends on stretching out of your own self and finding a sense of purpose. That might be political, it might be social, or it might be spiritual. This ain't always easy! At times, it's hard to know what you feel passionate about, what will make you feel great. Explore! Here are some ideas (and they're the tip of the iceberg):

✦ Find a cause to promote. World peace, animal rights, international workers' rights, rainforests, landmines— these are all issues that teens get involved with.

253

✧ Explore your spiritual side by joining a group at your church, temple, or mosque. Interested in other religions? Join a spiritual reading group at your local bookstore.

✧ Donate time to charity. Service to others can make you feel incredibly great.

✧ Start or join a literary club, an artist's collective, or a writing group. Actualize your creative side. There's far too little encouragement for the artist in us all.

Looking great comes from the inside. When you're directed, happy, and doing good things in the world, you'll look absolutely great doing them, too.

The Least You Need to Know

✧ Stress affects every aspect of your body and life.

✧ Exercise—as long as it's not obsessive—actually reduces stress.

✧ Teens need more sleep than other people. Get enough!

✧ You also can reduce stress through meditation, massage, and other nurturing activities.

✧ If it's more than stress, it might be a true depression, and you need to see a doctor.

Resources: Books, Magazines, and Cool Web Sites

Hey! This book is only a start. Here are some more resources—books, useful phone numbers, and Web sites—I've found that you can use to keep yourself looking and feeling great.

Really Great Books

Bell, Ruth. *Changing Bodies, Changing Lives*. Times Books, 1998.

Drill, Esther, Heather MacDonald, and Rebecca Odes. *Deal with It! A Whole New Approach to Your Body, Brain, and Life as a Gurl*. Pocket Books Trade Paperback, 1999. (Check out www.gurl.com, too!)

Lark, Dr. Susan. *Dr. Susan Lark's Premenstrual Syndrome Self-Help Book*. Celestial Arts, 1989.

Web Sites to Check Out

Here are some great Web sites for teens … about everything!

Fitness!

www.fitteen.com
Exercise and fitness site by and for teens.

Sex and Sexuality

www.teenwire.com
Planned Parenthood's teen site.

www.scarleteen.com
Real sex ed for real teens.

www.prematuree.com
Anonymous answers to life's embarrassing questions. Watch out. This site is graphic—it may even embarrass you!

Body Image

www.bodytalkmagazine.com
Positive body image and lifestyle issues.

www.about-face.org
Committed to changing the image of the ideal female body type.

Just Cool Stuff About Life

www.chickclick.com
www.stupidboy.com
The two sexes talking together.

www.hissyfit.com
Go here to rant and rave about your life.

www.goaskalice.columbia.edu
Answers about health, dating, sexuality, etc.

Self-Destructive Behavior and Eating Disorders

www.overeatersanonymous.org
For when your eating is out of control.

www.edrecovery.com
An online service providing info and programs to help you recover
from an eating disorder.

www.hugs.com
Info about a life without dieting.

www.selfharm.com
Info about self-harming behavior, support, and resources.

www.rocheford.org/suicide
Info about suicide, warning signs, and resources to help you.

Phone Numbers for Help and Guidance

Boys Town National Hotline
1-800-448-3000

Bilingual (English/Spanish) suicide hotline available 24/7 for everybody (not just boys).

KID SAVE
1-800-543-7283 (24 hours)

Info and referrals to shelters, substance-abuse treatment, mental-
health services, sexual-abuse treatment, and more, more, more.

Alanon-Alateen Information Service
1-800-344-2666

American Anorexia/Bulimia Association
212-891-8686

HIV/AIDS Hotline
1-800-342-AIDS

Planned Parenthood Federation of America
212-541-7800

SAFE (Self-Abuse Finally Ends)
1-800-DONT-CUT

STD Hotline
1-800-227-8922

Index

F

G

H–I

Check out
other
Complete Idiot's Guide® for Teens
Books

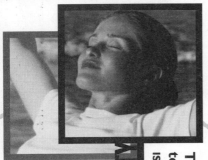

SPIRITUALITY

The Complete Idiot's Guide®
to Spirituality for Teens
ISBN: 002863926X

DATING

**The Complete Idiot's Guide®
to Dating for Teens**
ISBN: 0028639995

LOOKING GREAT

The Complete Idiot's Guide®
to Looking Great for Teens
ISBN: 0028639855

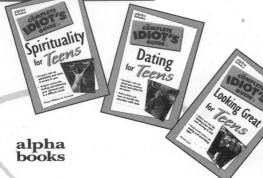

**alpha
books**